The HONEY
Prescription

The HONEY Prescription

The Amazing Power of Honey as Medicine

NATHANIEL ALTMAN

Healing Arts Press

Rochester, Vermont • Toronto, Canada

Healing Arts Press
One Park Street
Rochester, Vermont 05767
www.HealingArtsPress.com

Healing Arts Press is a division of Inner Traditions International

Note to the reader: *This book is intended as an informational guide. The remedies,
approaches, and techniques described herein are meant to supplement, and not to be a
substitute for, professional medical care or treatment. They should not be used to treat
a serious ailment without prior consultation with a qualified health care professional.*

Library of Congress Cataloging-in-Publication Data

The honey prescription : the amazing power of honey as medicine / Nathaniel
Altman.
    p. cm.
  Summary: "Explores the latest scientific research on the healing powers of
honey"—Provided by publisher.
  Includes bibliographical references and index.
  ISBN 978-1-59477-346-4
  1. Honey—Therapeutic use. I. Title.
  RM666.H55A48 2010
  615.8'54—dc22

                2009049324

Printed and bound in the United States by Lake Book Manufacturing

10   9   8   7   6   5   4   3   2   1

Text design by Jon Desautels and layout by Priscilla Baker
This book was typeset in Garamond Premier Pro with Parma Petit and Gill Sans
used as display typefaces

To send correspondence to the author of this book, mail a first-class letter to the
author c/o Inner Traditions • Bear & Company, One Park Street, Rochester, VT
05767, and we will forward the communication.

This book is dedicated with affection to my aunt and uncle, Mildred and Michael I. Aissen.

Disclaimer

The author of this book is not a physician. The following material is presented in the spirit of historical, philosophical, and scientific inquiry and is not offered as medical advice, diagnosis, or treatment of any kind. Those who wish to treat themselves with honey to cure a serious infection or other major health problem should do so only under the supervision of a qualified health care practitioner.

CONTENTS

ACKNOWLEDGMENTS

I would like to thank the following individuals for sending me copies of their research papers: Ali Al-Jabri, Joy Bardy, Shona Blair, Phil G. Bowler, Katrina Brudzynski, Neil Burton, Dee Carter, Rose Cooper, Ilteris Ensen, Jed W. Fahey, Peter Gallman, Ülkü Yapucu Günes, Ronald Ingle, Diane Langemo, Ahmad Mansour, Eraldo Medeiros Costa-Neto, Thangam Menon, Subramanian Natarajan, Aykut Misirlioglu, Rosa Ana Perez Martin, Faisal Rauf, Arne Simon, Peter Taormina, Alex Tonks, and Jenny Wilkinson.

I also thank the following for providing (and for permission to use) illustrations: The Town of Fahler, Alberta, for the "World's Biggest Bee" photo; Ronald Appleton of Appleton Galleries (Vancouver, BC) and Rupert Scow Jr. for permission to reproduce the photograph of Mr. Scow's wonderful Bee Mask, along with thanks to Sara Wark for taking the photo.

I would also like to thank the following members of my family and my friends for their encouragement, ideas, and support: Judith L. Aissen, Rudy Chapman, Edward Gasser, Mark E. Graboyes, Elizabeth and John Sell, Shi-Wei Shei, and Vincent Hsieh.

I am grateful to my literary agent, Stephany Evans of FinePrint Literary Management in New York City, who inspired me to write this book, for her continuous support and suggestions during its preparation.

Finally, special thanks go to Dr. Peter C. Molan, director of the

Honey Research Unit at the University of Waikato in New Zealand, for his generosity in supplying me with research material and for his many hours of consultation and advice.

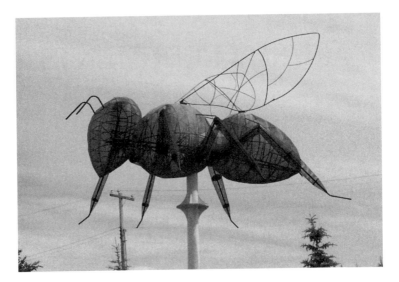

World's biggest bee. Photo courtesy of the Town of Fahler (Alberta, Canada).

INTRODUCTION

Like many people, I'm fascinated by honeybees and have been since childhood. I grew up on a three-acre "rocky farm" in upstate New York, with early memories of a rustic beehive that the previous owners attached to an old locust tree at the edge of our property. Every spring the bees would leave the hive and visit the blossoming peach trees, apple trees, and blackberry bushes on the hill behind our farmhouse. We also found them taking nectar from the forsythia, lilac, and rose bushes that bloomed in the yard. Like most boys raised in the country, my brother and I built lookouts and forts and often hiked through the property, where invariably we'd cross paths with bees and wasps. Yet unlike the wasps and yellow jackets that would often pursue and sometimes sting us, the honeybees tended to go about their business and left us alone.

Over the years I have written a number of books about natural and alternative healing, and my book *The Oxygen Prescription* (Healing Arts Press, 2007) focused on the therapeutic value of ozone and hydrogen peroxide. Our body naturally produces small amounts of hydrogen peroxide to help protect us from disease. Hydrogen peroxide not only helps oxygenate the body but also has the capacity to stimulate oxidative enzymes or proteins that accelerate oxidative reactions. They, in turn, can destroy viruses and bacteria. This is one reason why physicians have clinically administered small amounts of hydrogen peroxide (usually diluted in a standard saline solution) to patients as a healing agent for more than a hundred years.

I was surprised to learn that honey contains an enzyme that can

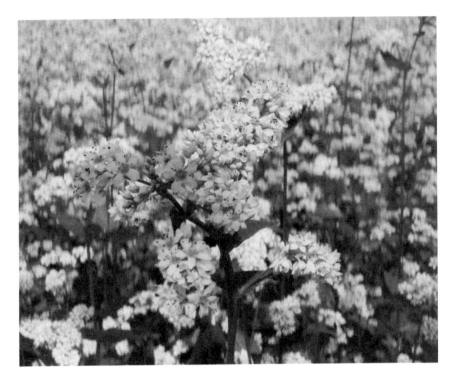

Buckwheat field. Photo by Hideo Sakata.

actually help produce low yet continuous levels of hydrogen peroxide. This has been found to be a major reason for honey's legendary ability to kill bacteria, viruses, and fungi.

The use of honey as a healing agent is nothing new. It was an ingredient in medicinal compounds and cures made by Egyptian physicians five thousand years ago. In India ayurvedic physicians recommended using honey to promote good health, while the ancient Greeks believed that honey could promote both virility and longevity. Traditional Chinese healers started using honey thousands of years ago, and it continues to make up an important part of Chinese medicine today.

Although several hundred articles on the medicinal value of honey appeared in medical and scientific journals between 1935 and 1990, scientific research was often overlooked by physicians who focused on antibiotics, antivirals, and other drugs to treat human disease.

But with the rapidly increasing spread of superbugs like methicillin-resistant *Staphylococcus aureus* (MRSA), vancomycin-resistant enterococci (VRE), various strains of extended-spectrum beta-lactamases (ESBLs), and other microbes like *Pseudomonas* and coagulase-negative staphylococci that are becoming resistant to antibiotics, modern medicine has taken a second look at the healing properties of honey.

- Scientists have found that honey has a powerful inhibitory effect on no fewer than sixty species of bacteria. Many of these bacteria are notoriously resistant to antibiotics, but they are powerless against the antibacterial properties of honey.
- Laboratory and clinical research has found that in addition to treating wounds and skin infections, honey can be useful for treating burns as well as a wide variety of internal diseases, including upper respiratory infections, cough, and intestinal disorders. Honey may even help control diabetes, calm the nerves, and even promote more restful sleep.
- Honey is becoming a popular ingredient in government-approved therapeutic salves, ointments, lozenges, and wound dressings.
- Unlike antibiotics and other medications, honey is nontoxic and produces no adverse side effects. It is also inexpensive, easy to obtain, and can be used by virtually anyone.

Yet the story of the therapeutic value of honey is invariably connected with the amazing creature that produces it, the honeybee. Human beings have exploited honeybees since pre-Egyptian times. Honey hunting and beekeeping are among the oldest and most widespread of human activities. Yet the current methods of industrial agriculture—where animals, plants, and the land that sustains them are treated as disposable commodities designed to return the greatest profit for the investment—pose a threat to the future well-being of bees, especially in North America, Europe, and other developed nations of the world.

While most of us think that bees are valued primarily as honey producers, their most important commercial value is that of pollinator. Honeybees pollinate most of the fruits and vegetables we eat: if it were not for their labor, these foods would never grow. The welfare of the honeybee and other insect pollinators is essential to our future well-being.

Writing *The Honey Prescription* has been an adventure. The original outline for the book contained fewer than ten chapters, and it was difficult to believe that there would be enough material to create a book with more than a hundred pages. As I proceeded to develop this project, I was amazed at the vast amount of articles about the healing properties of honey in scientific and medical journals, although most of the studies were done outside the United States. Much of this cutting-edge research will be presented for the first time to the general reader in this book. As I encountered more material about honey, new chapters took shape, and the book soon grew to more than twice its original size.

In addition to locating and studying hundreds of scientific papers in medical libraries and on the Internet as well as from many of the authors themselves, I had the honor of meeting Dr. Peter C. Molan, director of the Honey Research Unit at the University of Waikato in New Zealand. Although probably one of the busiest men in the country, he gave me a full day of his valuable time and patiently responded to dozens of questions that he'd probably answered many times before. Dr. Molan also gave me a sheaf of his dozens of scientific papers and offered tips on how to locate more information about therapeutic honey. He also gave me the "Grand Tour" of the laboratory of the Honey Research Unit, a unique research facility where many of the most exciting discoveries about honey's healing properties are taking place. I left the University of Waikato exhausted but inspired—far more aware of the complexities involved in honey research as well as the tremendous value of honey as a healing agent.

During the New Zealand trip, it was also possible to visit the impressive modern facilities of Comvita, located in the middle of kiwi-fruit orchards about a half-hour drive south of the city of Tauranga. A pioneer in the research and development of manuka honey health products, Comvita produces a variety of honey-based salves and dressings that are being used in leading hospitals in Europe and North America. I also had the pleasure of meeting Margaret Bennett, who, with her husband Bill, founded SummerGlow, one of New Zealand's most respected apiaries specializing in high-activity UMF-grade manuka honey and related products.

I believe that *The Honey Prescription* is the most complete and authoritative book of its kind to address the wide spectrum of medicinal uses of honey for both the general reader and health care practitioner. Drawing on centuries of material from historical, mythological, and folk-medicine sources from around the world, *The Honey Prescription* presents and evaluates the very latest in scientific and medical evidence of the healing properties of honey, often for the first time in book form. There are also extensive selections of honey-based recipes for both health and beauty, as well as a guide for locating the finest honey products available today.

At a time when health care consumers are looking for inexpensive, nontoxic, and effective remedies for both preventive care and to treat injury and illness, honey is a viable alternative to antibiotics and other medications. I hope that this book will stimulate discussion. I hope that this book will lead both the general public and members of the health care community to take a more serious look at the therapeutic potentials of honey. As a result, we can make more educated and intelligent decisions about the health care options available for ourselves and our families.

PART I

Grounding

I

WHO ARE THE HONEYBEES?

This tiny creature's achievements tower above the flights of architecture and efficiency of man-made machinery. It has occupied the minds of scientists, writers, musicians, and philosophers around the globe.

HATTIE ELLIS IN *SWEETNESS & LIGHT*

The honeybee (*Apis mellifera*) is one of nature's most magnificent and hardest working creatures. The most studied living being on the planet after humans, the honeybee has been called "the summit of sophisticated engineering" and "an evolutionary triumph of form and function in a thousand details." The result of millions of years of ever-growing perfection, the honeybee lives in perennial social societies that are a model of efficiency and cooperation.

Although domesticated and maintained in artificial hives throughout the world, the honeybee can build and sustain colonies of more than one hundred thousand individual members, all working together seamlessly for the good of the community. As the world's supreme pollinator of flowers, trees, and other plants, the honeybee allows the planet's land animals (including humans) to survive and thrive (figure 1.1).

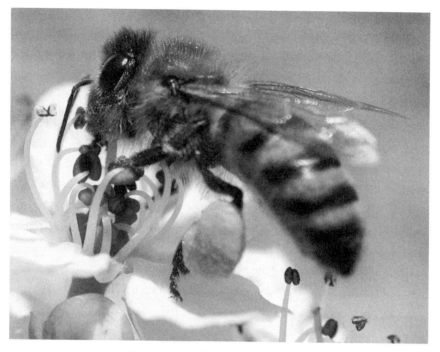

Figure 1.1. A honeybee on a flower

Honeybee Anatomy

When we watch a honeybee land on a flower, what do we see? A small but perfectly proportioned fluffy insect with large eyes, four slender wings, and a large tail with horizontal stripes.

A closer look reveals that this amazing insect's articulated body is covered with tiny hairs, including the eyes. Not only do the hairs create an electromagnetic charge that draws in pollen, but also the bristles of the eye (they are located between the 6,900 hexagonal plates or lenses that make up the eye) help the bee to gauge wind direction. The fine hairs on the forelegs allow the bee to clean its antennae, while those on the hind legs enable the bee to scoop pollen from the flower.

The body of the honeybee shares much in common with other insects: as opposed to an internal skeleton like vertebrates, it has a hard outer covering called an exoskeleton. The exoskeleton's job is to protect the bee's internal organs and to prevent its body from drying out.

Like other insects, honeybees have three body regions: the head, thorax, and abdomen. The head is composed of the sensory organs and appendages for ingestion like the mouth. The legs and wings are found on the thorax. The digestive and reproductive organs are located in the bee's abdomen. Let's take a closer look at this tiny (two-fifths to three-fifths of an inch [5 mm–15 mm]) marvel of engineering and efficiency. (See figure 1.2.)

The Head

When viewed from the front, the honeybee's head is triangular in shape. The two antennae are located close together near the center of the face. The bee has two compound eyes and three simple eyes, also located on the head. The honeybee uses its proboscis—a long hairy tongue—to feed on liquids like nectar. Its mandibles—described later on—are used to eat pollen and to fashion wax when building the honeycomb.

The honeybee's segmented antennae serve as important sensory organs. They are connected to the brain by a large double nerve that

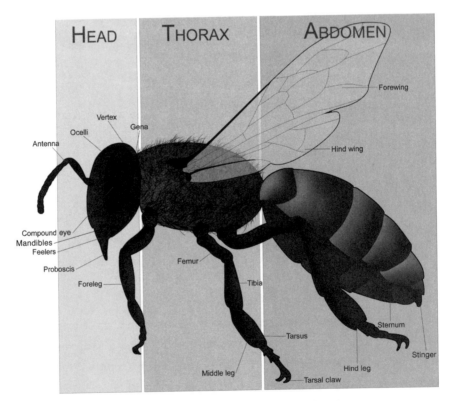

Figure 1.2. Anatomy of the honeybee

transmits all the important sensory information the honeybee receives to the brain. The tiny sensory hairs found on each antenna are highly responsive to odor and touch.

Honeybees have large compound eyes made up of almost seven thousand tiny lenses. Each lens takes in one small part of the bee's total vision. The brain then takes the image from each lens and creates one large mosaic-like picture, not unlike what happens when a television screen creates a picture out of millions of tiny dots. In addition to these two large compound eyes, honeybees have three smaller (and simpler) eyes called ocelli. They are located above the compound eyes. While the ocelli are sensitive to light, they cannot view images like the compound eyes can.

The honeybee's proboscis is essentially a long, slender, hairy tongue. This amazing tool works like a straw to suck liquid food (like nectar, honey, and water) into the female worker bee's mouth. After feeding, she simply draws up the proboscis and folds it behind her head.

The honeybee has a pair of mandibles that are like pliers. Located on either side of the head, they are used for any job that calls for grasping or cutting: working the wax in honeycomb construction, squeezing flower parts (anthers) to release pollen, carrying refuse out of the hive, or gripping intruders when the bees defend their home.

The Thorax

The thorax is the middle part of the bee and where the three pairs of legs and two pairs of wings are attached.

The honeybee has three pairs of segmented legs that are used primarily for walking. However, the forelegs have tiny hairs designed to clean the antennae and keep them sensitive; the hind legs contain pollen baskets. The surface of the outer hind leg is fringed with long, curved hairs that hold the pollen in place. This enclosed space is used to carry pollen from the flowers back to the hive. Once the bees have gathered the pollen, they move it to the "pollen press" located between the two largest segments of the hind leg. It is used to press the pollen into pellets.

The honeybee has two pairs of flat, thin, membranous wings. The front wings are bigger than the hind wings, but the two wings on each side work together in flight. An aerodynamic wonder, the bee's ability to fly is not just from the opposite sets of wings flapping but from a propeller-like twist given to each wing (on the same side) during the upstroke and the downstroke. These light, efficient, and powerful wings produce approximately 230 beats per second or 13,800 beats a minute.

The Abdomen

The honeybee's abdomen is made up of nine segments. The wax and some scent glands are located in these nine segments, while the stinger is found in a pocket at the tapered end.

The worker honeybee has eight specialized wax glands. The wax produced by these glands is discharged as a liquid, which is stored in specialized pockets while it hardens into small flakes or scales. The worker bee removes the wax scales with a special comb located on the inside hind leg. She then transfers the wax scale to her mandibles, where she chews the wax until it becomes a compact, pliant mass. The bee then adds the wax to the honeycomb.

The stinger is found at the end of the abdomen. It is similar to the egg-laying organ found in most other insects, except that it ejects venom instead of eggs. This is why only female bees can have a stinger. Hollow like a hypodermic needle, the stinger is about one-eighth of an inch (0.32 cm) long and is normally retracted within the abdomen. The tip is barbed so it can enter the victim's body easily but cannot be pulled out. In the struggle to free herself after the honeybee stings her victim, she leaves a portion of the stinger behind. The resulting damage is enough to kill her. The stinger continues to contract by reflex action, continuously pumping venom into the wound for several seconds.

Life in Honeybee Society

A colony of honeybees can contain between thirty and sixty thousand workers in early summer, plus a queen and up to three thousand drones, whose sole purpose is to mate with the single queen. The social life of the honeybee has always been viewed as a model of industry, cooperation, and efficiency. Each member of a bee community has a specific role in life and numerous tasks to accomplish. An old graphic depicting a beekeeper and a variety of bees is reproduced in figure 1.3.

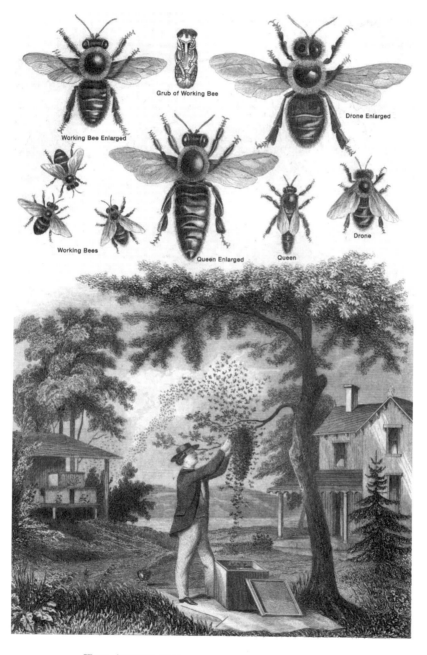

THE APIARY. THE BEE-KEEPER AT HIS WORK.

Figure 1.3. "The Apiary. The Bee-keeper at His Work"
depicts the various types of honeybee.

The Worker Bees

Most of the adult honeybees in a colony are female worker bees. They aren't called worker bees by accident, because they perform a wide range of jobs during the few short months from birth to death. As the ultimate multitasker, the worker bee's life includes:

- tending and feeding young bees, known as larvae;
- making honey;
- making royal jelly and beebread to feed larvae;
- producing wax;
- keeping the hive cool by fanning her wings;
- gathering and storing pollen, nectar, and water;
- guarding the hive from intruders;
- building, cleaning, and repairing the comb; and
- feeding and taking care of the queen and drones.

The life cycle of the worker bee passes through four distinct life stages: the egg, larva, pupa, and adult. The process is called complete metamorphosis, which means that the form of the bee changes drastically from the larva to the adult. A worker bee passes through the immature stages in about three weeks.

On the first day, the queen bee lays a single egg in each cell of the comb. The egg generally hatches into a larva on the fourth day. The larva is not a pretty sight: it is essentially a grub that resembles a tiny white sausage. The larva is fed a mixture of pollen and nectar called beebread. On the ninth day the cell is capped with wax, and the larva transforms into the pupa. The pupa is a physical transition stage between the amorphous larva and the winged adult. After three weeks the new adult worker bee is born. When born in the summer, a worker bee can live as long as three months.

The Drones' Life

The male members of the colony are known as drones. They are somewhat larger than worker bees and make up only about 5 percent of the hive population. Although they rarely survive longer than two months, the drones live a life of luxury. They don't collect pollen and cannot secrete royal jelly. They are totally supported by the female worker bees, who feed them with worker jelly. Drones have huge compound eyes, which meet at the top of the heads, plus have an extra segment in their antennae that helps them locate (and connect with) a flying queen. Like all other male bees and wasps, drones do not have stingers.

The Queen Bee

There is only one queen in a honeybee colony. Slightly larger than a worker bee, she has a longer abdomen. Eggs that are destined to become queens are laid in a larger cell, and the larvae are fed only royal jelly rather than ordinary beebread.

After she is born, the adult queen has only one job: to lay eggs. She can lay up to two thousand eggs a day. The queen is fed by the worker bees and never leaves the hive except to mate.

Queen bees also have stingers and use them in battles with each other so the winner can take over the colony. If a hapless new queen emerges from her incubation cell and is detected by the current queen, the reigning monarch will try her utmost to kill her rival. This is how the stability of the colony is maintained. When a queen gets old or weak and slows her production of queen substance—a perfumelike chemical signal called a pheromone that attracts the drones—she is generally replaced by a new queen. New queens are also produced in colonies about to swarm. A queen bee can live for up to five years, which is approximately fifty times longer than the average worker bee.

The Nuptial Flight

The virgin queen takes her nuptial flight sometime within the first week or two of her life. She flies out of the hive and begins to produce queen substance. There are many different types of pheromones that bees and other insects produce to direct or influence the behavior of other insects. The drones are strongly attracted to the specific "come hither" pheromone the queen produces, and those in the area soar skyward to try to connect with her and mate with her. The queen will mate with as many as twenty of them. Soon after mating, each drone dies.

The short life of the average drone is one of leisure with the possibility for sex. While the drone awaits the opportunity to mate with a virgin queen, he is fed royal jelly and otherwise cared for by the worker bees. On occasion, he may leave the hive to test his wings. Yet the drone's days are always numbered. If he mates with the queen, he dies. And if he doesn't mate with the queen, he is evicted from the hive by the same worker bees that fed and coddled him before the queen's nuptial flight, as seen in figure 1.4. Because his only talent is to mate with the queen, an evicted drone cannot fend for himself. He soon dies.

The Queen Mother

Once the queen has mated, she returns to the hive and starts laying eggs in chambers made of beeswax that the worker bees have built especially for this purpose. A queen can lay her own weight in eggs every day. She can also maintain the sperm she has collected for her lifetime in a special pouch in her body; as a result, she can lay eggs indefinitely. The fertilized eggs laid by a queen become female worker bees and new queens. The queen also lays some unfertilized eggs, which produce the drones.

The average queen bee lives for about a year-and-a-half, although some have been known to survive for up to six years. While she is alive and

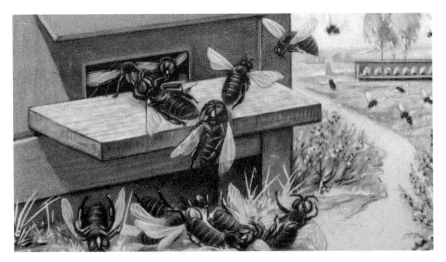

Figure 1.4. "The Eviction of the Drones" ("Le massacre").
From The Life of Bees, *The Liebig Company, 1932.*

active, the queen is constantly cared for by workers acting as attendants. If a queen dies prematurely and the colony had no new queen to replace her, the colony will eventually perish.

Saying Good-Bye

When the colony starts to become too crowded, some of the bees—along with the old queen—split off to form a new colony. This is called swarming. Before they leave, special preparations are made to ensure both the survival of the original hive and the bees that are starting the new colony: the eggs for new queens are laid in special larger cells and are carefully nurtured by remaining worker bees. Also, the departing bees engorge themselves on their honey reserves before leaving so as to have enough energy to make it to a new location.

Honeybee Memory

Because foraging is essential to the colony's survival, a worker bee must remember the color and shape of the different plants that contain pollen. It also needs to remember where they are and how to return to the hive after gathering the nectar and pollen. A study carried out at the Australian National University in Canberra found that even though the honeybee contains a tiny brain (it is just one millimeter in diameter and weighs about one milligram—just a hundredth of its body weight of 100 mg), it possesses a sophisticated memory. Honeybees not only plan their activities in a context of both time and space but also figure out what actions are to be performed at the appropriate time. They also have the capacity to synchronize their behavior with daily floral rhythms and forage when both nectar and pollen are at their highest levels. The researchers observed:

> Since the species of flowers that are in bloom, say, in the morning are more likely to be replaced by a different species at a different location in the afternoon, the bee needs, and has indeed evolved, an impressive ability to learn and memorize local features and routes, as well as the time of blooming, quickly and accurately.[1]

This amazing ability enables a bee that visits a particular manuka bush on Monday morning at 9 a.m., for example, to return to that same manuka bush the following morning at exactly the same time.

Bee Communication

When one lives in a small yet populated community, good communication is essential. Recent scientific evidence has shown that honeybees communicate in a variety of ways.

Pheromone Activity

I mentioned earlier that the queen bee attracts drones by releasing a type of chemical known as a pheromone. She produces other pheromones to help the community recognize her, to reduce the amount of egg laying by worker bees, and to keep the bees together when they form a new colony through swarming.

Worker bees also produce different types of pheromones to communicate with other bees in the hive. These pheromones can induce others to fan their wings to cool down the hive, to keep close to each other when they swarm, or to sound the alarm to protect the hive when an invader is near. When a bee stings a perceived invader, the venom attracts other bees, inducing them to sting in the exact same place.

The Waggle Dance

There are other methods of bee communication besides the one involving chemical pheromones. The best known is the "waggle dance": a unique, figure-eight dance through which a forager bee can share information with her hive mates about the direction of and distance to patches of flowers yielding nectar or pollen, or both. She can also direct them to important water sources.

First explained by the Austrian ethologist (a scientist who studies animal behavior) Karl von Frisch in *The Dance Language and Orientation of Bees* (The Belknap Press of Harvard University Press) in 1967, the waggle dance is a precise mechanism whereby successful foragers can recruit other members of the colony to good locations for collecting vital community resources.

According to the Carl Hayden Bee Research Center, a facility operated by the United States Department of Agriculture's Agricultural Research Service at the University of Arizona, the waggle dance involves a number of highly complex activities:

1. The forager bee or recruit locates a rich flower patch, imbibes some nectar, and flies home.
2. She crawls onto the vertical combs near the nest entrance and dances for up to several minutes.
3. The dance—performed amid closely packed adjacent bees—consists of running through a small figure-eight pattern repeatedly.
4. The figure-eight pattern is comprised of a straight run followed by a gradual turn to the right, after which the bee circles back to the starting point; another straight run, followed by a turn and circle to the left, and so on in a regular alternation.
5. The informative portion of the dance is the straight run, where the dancer vigorously vibrates (waggles) her abdomen back and forth laterally, emitting strong substrate and airborne vibrations. This is done in addition to buzzes that humans can hear.
6. The bee's flight muscles produce the buzzing sound. It has a frequency range between 200 and 300 cycles per second.
7. A new recruit may attend several such dances before she leaves the colony to locate food.
8. The direction and duration of straight runs are closely correlated with the direction and distance of the flower patch advertised by the dancing bee.
9. Flowers located directly in line with the sun are represented by waggle straight runs in an upward direction on the vertical combs, and any angle to the right or left of the sun's position is coded by a corresponding angle to the right or left of vertical. The angle between vertical and the straight waggling run of the dance is equal to the angle between the sun (its azimuth as opposed to its elevation above the horizon) and the flight direction from hive to food source.
10. The distance between the beehive and target plant appears to be encoded in the duration of the straight runs, since this is the feature

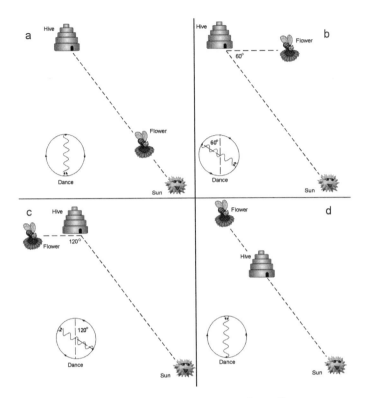

Figure 1.5. Four types of waggle dance. From the Bellarmine University Department of Biology, Louisville, Kentucky.

of the dance that exhibits the highest correlation with distance to the goal. The farther away the target, the longer the straight runs, with a rate of increase of about 75 milliseconds per 100 meters.[2]

In addition to these movements, dancing bees also communicate floral odors that cling to their setae and waxy cuticle. Four different types of waggle dance can be seen in figure 1.5.

How the Bees Make Honey

The major source of honey is nectar from flowers, but in some forest areas, honeydew can be the primary source. Honeydew comes from the excretions of insects that suck the sap of plants.

Unlike the message "Flowers make honey" in the charming old

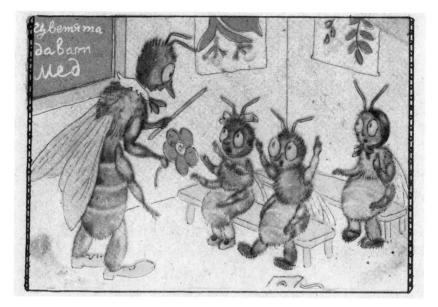

Figure 1.6. Lesson for young bees: "flowers make honey." A vintage Bulgarian postcard, date unknown.

Bulgarian postcard (reproduced in figure 1.6), the flowers provide most of the raw materials that bees use to create this unique product. First, plants produce nectar to attract bees and other insects. Pollen is also trapped in nectar that is collected by bees: the pollen comes from the anthers of the flowers that are producing the nectar.

Both the bee and the flower are perfectly suited for each other: the pollen is designed to become attached to the insect, and the hairs on the bee's body are perfectly designed to attract it. The bee actually wallows in the flower, completely dusting itself with pollen. The pollen is then carried to another flower of the same species, which increases the flower's chance of being pollinated.

From the bee's point of view, pollen is an important source of protein, vitamins, minerals, and fats for the honeybee colony. It is collected by the bee and packed into the honey sacks on her hind legs. At the same time, the honeybee sucks the nectar from the flower and stores it in her stomach. Saliva is added from the bee's salivary and hypopharyngeal glands, which begin the process of converting the nectar into honey. When she has found all the pollen and nectar she can carry, she returns to the hive.

Upon returning to the hive, the bee regurgitates the nectar, passing it on to the house bees who add their own saliva to the liquid. At the same time, they draw the converted nectar out on their tongue to allow the water in the honey to evaporate. When the water content drops to 35 to 40 percent (from the original 60–75 percent) the bees spread the sweet liquid onto the walls of the hexagonal-shaped cells of their honeycomb and continue to fan it with their wings. This will help evaporate the excess water and prevent the solution from fermenting.

The honey will gradually cure over several days of constant fanning. The worker bees regulate the temperature of the hive between 82.4° and 95°F (28° and 35°C) to assist in the curing process. When the water content of the honey drops below 20 percent, they seal the top of the cell with wax that comes from special wax glands on the underside of their abdomens. The enzymes added by the bees during the earlier honey-making process continue to ripen the honey while it is stored.

A Lifetime of Effort

For the bees, the production of honey is truly a lifetime effort. Here are a few random facts:

- It takes nectar from approximately 2.6 million flowers to make one pound of honey (more than 5.7 million flowers for 1 kilogram).
- Depending on the flower source, a honeybee must visit between several hundred to more than one thousand flowers in order to fill her honey stomach.
- A colony of bees may collectively travel as far as fifty-five thousand miles to make just a pound of honey.
- It takes one thousand bees to make a mere ounce of honey. This is more than a single honeybee can produce in its entire life.
- A hive can produce sixty to one hundred pounds of honey a year.
- A bee colony of one hundred thousand bees can make ten pounds of honey per day, which is much more than the bees need themselves. They usually produce about one hundred extra pounds per summer.

- In the United States, the yearly per capita consumption of all sweeteners (including cane sugar; high-fructose corn syrup; high-intensity, low-calorie sweeteners like aspartame; and honey) exceeds 170 pounds (77.2 kilograms). U.S. per capita consumption of honey alone is around 1.3 pounds (0.59 kg) a year.

Extracting the Honey

A super is the part of a commercial beehive that is used to collect honey. Honey supers may contain eight to ten frames where the bees live and maintain their honeycomb. The most common variety has a depth of 6⅝ inches (approximately 14 cm). During a honey flow beekeepers may put several honey supers onto a hive so the bees have enough storage space.

Because bees understandably do not want their honey to be removed, the beekeeper is often in danger of getting stung. He or she (most bee-keepers happen to be male) use either a brush soaked with water to brush the bees off the honeycombed frame (the water makes their wings too heavy to fly) or smoke, which is believed to quiet down the bees. Wise beekeepers do not take all of the honey: they leave enough for the bees to feed on during the winter. A minority of commercial beekeepers simply kills the bees outright and takes all the honey.

Although some honey is sold in the form of honeycomb, most is extracted from the comb before marketing. Once removed from the hive, the honeycomb cappings are stripped off the frames with a hot electric knife. The cappings are later collected and melted down to get the wax, which can then be used for sealing preserves or making candles.

The uncapped frames are then placed in an extractor, which resembles an old-fashioned washing machine drum activated by a pulley that spins the frames around. Honey is sprayed out of the frames and drips down the inside of a drum to collect at the bottom. Each frame is spun first with one side outward, then flipped to expose the other side. The empty frames—known as stickies—are then returned to the hive.

2

HONEY:
GIFT OF THE GODS

Honey is a wonderful gift of nature, and stands almost
alone as a pure natural sweet, perfect in itself.

SAMUEL SIMMINS, *A MODERN BEE FARM*
AND ITS ECONOMIC MANAGEMENT, 1887

The remarkable honeybee makes a remarkable product. Treasured for more than ten thousand years, the use of honey parallels the evolution of human society. It has been used as a source of food by nearly every culture, and it has also been a part of religious and healing ceremonies in many corners of the world. Until recently, honey was one of the only concentrated forms of sugar available in most parts of the world. The same cultural richness has produced an equally colorful variety of uses of honey in other products ranging from cake to medicine to cosmetics.

Honey: The Definition

What is honey? A reliable definition can be found in the Codex Alimentarius—or food code—that was developed by the United Nations Food and Agriculture Organization. It is the global reference for commercial food producers, food processors, and national food control agencies around the world. In 2001 it offered the following general definition of honey in which all commercially required characteristics of the product are described.

> Honey is the natural sweet substance produced by honey bees from the nectar of plants or from secretions of living parts of plants or excretions of plant sucking insects on the living parts of plants, which the bees collect, transform by combining with specific substances of their own, deposit, dehydrate, store and leave in the honey comb to ripen and mature.[1]

Honey: Two Basic Types

I mentioned earlier that there are several hundred species of bees that produce honey, and other types of bees and even wasps are known to store different kinds of honey as food reserves. Yet because the vast majority of the honey we consume today is produced by one bee species, known as *Apis mellifera,* any references to honey made in this book will refer to this species unless otherwise specified. The codex provides two further definitions of honey produced by *Apis mellifera.*

1. Blossom honey or nectar honey is distinguished as coming from the nectaries of flowers, or the plant glands that secrete a sweet substance called nectar. The vast majority of honey we consume is blossom honey.
2. Honeydew honey comes from the excretions of insects—such as aphids, whiteflies, mealybugs, and other sapsuckers—that suck the sap of plants. In Europe the major source of honeydew is evergreen trees, and the final product is often marketed as forest honey.

While popular in some European countries and other areas of the world, beekeepers often find it difficult to sell forest honey because it has a stronger flavor than blossom honey. Very often, bees collecting this resource have to be fed protein supplements, because honeydew lacks the protein-rich pollen that is gathered from flowers.

Honey Purity

In addition, the codex states that honey sold to the public is not to be adulterated with extenders like water or any type of sugar or syrup. This includes primarily high-fructose corn syrup routinely used by the food-processing industry to sweeten cereals, breads, pastries, and processed fruits and vegetables.

> Honey sold as such shall not have added to it any food ingredient, including food additives, nor shall any other additions be made other than honey. Honey shall not have any objectionable matter, flavour, aroma, or taint absorbed from any foreign matter during its processing and storage.[2]

In the chapter he wrote for the textbook *Food Authentication,* Dr. Peter C. Molan, director of the Honey Research Unit at the University of Waikato in New Zealand, referred to adulteration of honey as a "major problem," citing that "the extent to which this happens is great enough to cause serious concerns to apiarists, leading to them taking action at attempt to stop the practice."[3]

China has been a major source of adulterated honey. According to a 2007 report by S. Kamberg & Company, Ltd., a leading international food broker,

> The USA had previously been receiving a lot of packer's syrup from China (honey blended with other sugar syrups). It is uncertain if this was actual packer's syrup, or possibly actual honey sold as packer's syrup to avoid duties. The probability is high that any actual packer's syrup entering this country would be blended with and sold as real honey.[4]

Adulteration of honey in China has been an ongoing problem for decades. The Chinese government and industry groups like the China Bee Products Association (CBPA) have been working with producers and exporters to improve the quality of honey sold domestically and abroad.

Honey Composition

Honey is one of the most complex natural foods available today and contains a wide variety of nutrients. Although darker honeys tend to provide higher amounts of minerals than lighter varieties, 100 grams (about 5 tablespoons) of honey contain approximately 304 calories and average 17.1 grams of water, with a range of 12.2 to 22.9 grams.[5]

According to the National Honey Board, which represents the honey industry in the United States, honey averages 82.4 percent carbohydrate. Based on 100 grams, that includes 38.5 grams of fructose, 31 grams of glucose, 7.2 grams of maltose, and just over 1 gram of sucrose.

Fructose and glucose are monosaccharides, or simple sugars, while sucrose is a disaccharide with fructose and glucose linked together. Honey also contains more complex carbohydrates known as oligosaccharides, which are medium-size carbohydrates containing more than three simple sugar subunits, often made up of mono- and disaccharides. These sugars are formed when nectar and honeydew are converted to honey. Oligosaccharides are sometimes referred to as higher sugars. As we'll see later on, they encourage the growth of "friendly bacteria" in the intestinal tract, which has been found to contribute to good health.

Even though honey contains an average of only 0.5 percent protein, amino acids, vitamins, and minerals, it has more nutrients than refined sugars like table sugar and corn syrup. In addition, the body easily assimilates these trace amounts. When added together, they are considered a valuable source of nutrition. Vitamins include thiamin, riboflavin, niacin, pantothenic acid, pyridoxine, and ascorbic acid (vitamin C), while the most important minerals include calcium, copper, iron, magnesium, manganese, phosphorus, potassium, chromium, selenium, and zinc.[6]

The "Extras"

Over the past ten years researchers from around the world have found that in addition to these nutrients, honey contains several highly beneficial elements—pre- and probiotics—that make it an important nutritional and medicinal resource.

Pre- and Probiotics

Pre- and probiotics make up a group of friendly bacteria considered important to the health of the gastrointestinal tract. Although all honey is naturally antibacterial, I mentioned earlier that it contains a variety of oligosaccharides. These complex sugars may function as prebiotic. Research conducted at Michigan State University found that adding honey to fermented dairy products like yogurt can enhance the growth of friendly bacteria.[7]

Antioxidant Activity

As we'll see later on, honey has been found to contain a variety of flavonoids and phenolic acids that act as antioxidants whose job is to scavenge and eliminate free radicals. Research has shown that by consuming more antioxidant-rich foods, we may be able to help protect our bodies from cellular damage and possibly delay the aging process and the development of degenerative diseases like cancer, heart disease, and diabetes.

The amount and type of these antioxidant compounds in honey depends largely on the floral source. Generally speaking, darker honeys (such as buckwheat and lavender) possess higher antioxidant activity than lighter varieties like fireweed and acacia.[8]

When compared to antioxidant-containing foods like oranges, broccoli, spinach, sweet potatoes, tomatoes, and green tea, the antioxidant content of honey is small. However researchers at the University of Illinois—who compared the antioxidant value of different foods—concluded:

> While this comparison demonstrates that honey may not serve as a major source of dietary antioxidants, it nonetheless demonstrates the potential for honey to play an important (and as yet unrealized) role in providing antioxidants in a highly palatable form . . . certain unifloral honeys may thus make a unique contribution as a palatable supplementary source of plant antioxidants, particularly if used to replace sucrose, which has no antioxidant value, in the diet.[9]

Hydrogen Peroxide Activity

The antibacterial activity of honey is usually due to the production of small amounts of hydrogen peroxide, a clear, colorless liquid that easily mixes with water. Known chemically as H_2O_2, it is a compound made up of two hydrogen atoms and two oxygen atoms. Hydrogen peroxide is normally created in the atmosphere when ultraviolet light strikes oxygen in the presence of moisture. Hydrogen peroxide reacts easily with other substances and is able to kill bacteria, fungi, parasites, viruses, and some types of tumor cells. The first medical use of hydrogen peroxide was reported in *The Journal of the American Medical Association* in 1888 and—along with therapeutic ozone and hyperbaric oxygen—has become a part of a group of a healing modality generally known as oxidative therapy or oxygen therapy.[10]

Hydrogen peroxide occurs naturally within Earth's biosphere, and traces of it are found in rain and snow. It has also been found in many of the healing springs of the world, including Fátima in Portugal, Lourdes in France, and the Shrine of St. Anne in Québec. Hydrogen peroxide is also an important component of plant life, and small amounts are found in many vegetables and fruits, including fresh cabbage, tomatoes, asparagus, green peppers, watercress, oranges, apples, and watermelons.

When honey comes into contact with body fluids like saliva or moisture (exudate) produced by a wound, an enzyme known as glucose oxidase (introduced into the honey by the bee) slowly releases hydrogen peroxide, often in sufficient amounts to be effective against bacteria. The production of H_2O_2 is a major reason why honey can kill an astonishing variety of bacteria and viruses, including "superbugs" like *Pseudomonas aeruginosa* and MRSA.[11] However, levels of H_2O_2 remain well below the level that causes inflammatory effects.

Yet glucose oxidase can be destroyed when honey is exposed to light or heat, which will stop the production of hydrogen peroxide. That is the main reason why honey should be stored in a cool place, kept away from sunlight, and consumed at temperatures under 100°F (38°C).

Non–Hydrogen Peroxide Antibacterial Activity

Some honeys do not possess hydrogen peroxide but contain phytochemicals—chemical compounds derived from plants or fruits—that have strong antibacterial activity. The most important of these include certain types of manuka honey, made from the flowers of the *Leptospermum* plant, which grows uncultivated in different regions of Australia and New Zealand. For this reason, honey from Leptospermum—especially manuka honey in New Zealand—has been the focus of dozens of scientific studies and clinical trials. It has also been the only honey used in government-approved medical creams and wound dressings marketed to hospitals and physicians around the world.

Active manuka honey is the only honey available for sale that is tested for its antibacterial activity. This activity is called the Unique Manuka Factor (UMF).* The presence of this activity can be detected by laboratory testing, a process developed by the Honey Research Unit at the University of Waikato in Hamilton, New Zealand. Honey that is tested and verified to have a level of ten or more is given a UMF rating and is referred to as "active." UMF-rated New Zealand manuka honey is considered the top medicinal honey in the world. Active UMF-rated honey must comply with the following five criteria:

1. It has the trademark UMF clearly stated on the front label.
2. It is packed into jars and labeled in New Zealand.
3. It is supplied from a New Zealand licensee that is licensed to use the trademark UMF.
4. It has the UMF licensee's name and license number on the label.
5. It has a UMF rating as a number on the label. The higher the number, the greater the UMF test result and corresponding antimicrobial, therapeutic, and healing qualities.

---

*As mentioned in the numbered list, the term "UMF" is a trademarked by the Active Manuka Honey Association. Throughout the text the trademark symbol will not be repeated but should be assumed by the reader. For more details about the association and the process of determining UMF ratings, see the "Power of Manuka" section in chapter 5.

Certified Active UMF-Manuka honey carries the UMF trademark on the label (as seen on the two jars of Active UMF-Manuka honey in figure 2.1) plus a license number on the side or back. If these are absent, the honey is of dubious medicinal value and should be avoided. I will discuss the scientific basis of the healing power of manuka honey and more about its rating system in chapter 5.

On the Market

Many honey aficionados have compared it to wine. Like wine, there are hundreds of honey types. Even the same type of honey can vary tremendously. Some of the determining factors include climate, amount of rainfall, soil composition, the time the honey is collected, ambient temperature, and the level of care involved in harvesting and packing. The result is a huge variety of honeys of different colors, tastes, aromas, and textures. Like the finest wines, some honey is extremely rare and can cost

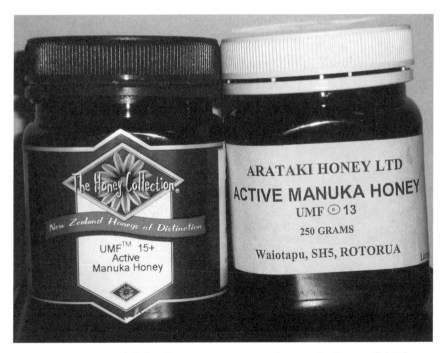

Figure 2.1. Two labels of genuine UMF-rated Manuka honey. (L) The Honey Collection, for both domestic use and export; (R) Arataki honey, sold for domestic use. Photo by Nathaniel Altman.

more than $200 a pound. And like cheap wine, some honeys are essentially "utility grade" and are sold in bulk to manufacturers of breakfast cereals and to large bakery operators.

Most honey comes from bees foraging on several different floral sources: these honeys are known as polifloral. Yet some early- or late-blooming plants provide enough nectar during a short growing season, so a colony can yield honey from a single type of flower. Although rarely found, purely monofloral honeys are especially prized by beekeepers and honey connoisseurs alike. Most of the honey marketed as "monofloral" may in fact contain a majority of honey from the particular flower but is allowed to contain small amounts of honey from other flower species.

Each type of honey has a distinct aroma, flavor, and color depending on the individual floral source as well as the region from where it is harvested. Some honeys mimic the unique characteristics of the flower that the honeybee has visited, such as orange blossom, rosemary, thyme, or buckwheat. A listing and description of some the world's most popular honeys can be found in the appendix.

While there are literally hundreds of varieties of honey, there are nine basic types sold in supermarkets, farm stands, apiaries, gourmet food shops, and natural food stores as well as from online suppliers.

Comb Honey

Comb honey is honey that comes in the honeybees' wax comb (figure 2.2, upper right). Both the comb and the honey are edible. It is often packaged by installing a wooden framework in special honey supers, and the honey is then cut from the wooden frames. It generally costs more than liquid honey sold in a bottle.

Cut Comb Honey

Cut comb honey is liquid honey that has added chunks of the honeycomb in the jar. It's also known as "liquid–cut comb combination."

Liquid Honey

Liquid honey is free of visible crystals and is extracted from the honeycomb by centrifugal force, gravity, or straining. Because this type of honey

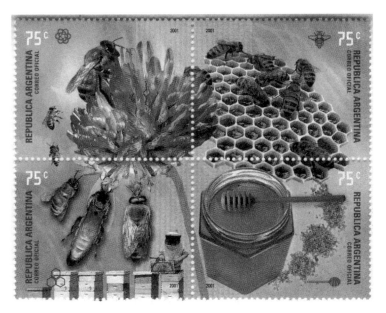

Figure 2.2. Bees and honey; from a set of Argentine postage stamps

mixes easily into a variety of foods, it's very popular for cooking and baking. Most of the honey consumed in the United States and Canada is sold in liquid form.

Naturally Crystallized Honey

Honey is sometimes sold in a semisolid state known as crystallized or granulated honey. This natural phenomenon takes place when glucose, one of three main sugars in honey, spontaneously precipitates out of the supersaturated honey solution. The glucose loses water (becoming glucose monohydrate) and takes the form of a crystal, defined as a solid body with a precise and orderly structure. The crystals form a type of lattice that immobilizes other components of honey and keeps them in suspension. This is why it takes on a semisolid state.

Although honey will not spoil, nearly all types of honey will naturally crystallize over time. Even though some people buy and consume their honey in crystallized form, others prefer to use it as a liquid. If you want to liquefy crystallized honey, place the honey jar in warm water and stir until the crystals dissolve.

Whipped Honey

Like naturally crystallized honey, whipped honey (also known as creamed honey) is also sold in a crystallized state. However, the crystallization is controlled so that, at room temperature, the honey can be easily spread like butter. In many countries around the world, whipped honey is preferred to the liquid form, because it is easier to use on bread.

Raw Honey

Raw honey is honey in the form as it exists in the beehive or as obtained by extraction, settling, or straining without adding heat above 120°F (48.0°C).

Raw honey usually carries some traces of pollen and may contain small particles of wax. Local raw honey is popular with allergy sufferers because the pollen impurities are thought to reduce sensitivity to hay fever.

Filtered Honey

Also known as strained honey, filtered honey has been passed through a mesh material to remove particulate material, such as pieces of wax and propolis, without removing pollen. It often has a cloudy appearance due to the remaining pollen.

Ultrafiltered Honey

Ultrafiltered honey is the kind usually sold in supermarkets. Unlike raw or filtered honey, it is processed by very fine filtration under high pressure

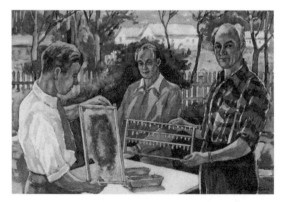

Figure 2.3. An old German postcard depicting a group
of men examining honeycomb at market

to remove all extraneous solids and pollen grains. The process typically requires heating the honey to 150°F to 170°F (65°C–77°C) to allow it to more easily pass through the fine filter, which leaves it very clear. Grocers like this type of honey because it crystallizes more slowly and thus has a longer shelf life.

The major downside to ultrafiltration is that it eliminates nutritionally valuable enzymes found in raw honey, such as diastase and invertase. While it does not affect either the honey's taste or nutritional value, heating destroys hydrogen peroxide activity, a natural component of raw, unprocessed honey. Hydrogen peroxide is one of the major elements that makes honey a powerful antibacterial agent and healer.

Certified Organic Honey

Organic honey is certified to be free of pesticides and antibiotics by the United States Department of Agriculture (USDA) and a USDA certified or recognized organization like the Global Organic Alliance. In Canada organic products carry a logo of the Canadian General Standards Board, while in New Zealand, NZ Organic is certified by AgriQuality and BioGro NZ. Other countries have their own certifying agencies.

How can honey be organic? First, the beehives are specifically placed in isolated areas away from any type of contamination, such as golf courses, agricultural areas, heavy traffic areas, and landfills.

Second, the bees' natural instinct governs their flying range. It tells them to stay within approximately a two-mile (3.2 kilometer) radius from their hive. Their uncanny sense of direction allows them to return to their hive without delay: this phenomenon is probably the origin of the term "making a beeline." Yet when the bees fly beyond this designated range, all sense of direction is lost.

As can be imagined, organic honey is quite rare. Most commercial beekeepers routinely use sulfa compounds and antibiotics to control bee diseases and carbolic acid to remove honey from the hive. Although most small-scale beekeepers do not kill their bees and leave enough honey for the colony to survive, large-scale beekeepers tend to take all the honey and provide their bees with substitute foods like high-fructose corn syrup or more nutritional supplements. A minority of beekeepers uses calcium cyanide to kill colonies before extracting the honey. In many parts of the world, conventional honeybees gather nectar from plants that have been sprayed with pesticides.

Where Does Your Honey Come From?

In addition, some bee colonies—especially in China—are located in industrial zones or other areas with considerable air pollution. This can lead to contamination of the honey with noxious or toxic chemicals.

In the Ukraine, Russia, and Belarus the nuclear reactor disaster at Chernobyl in 1986 polluted parts of these countries with radioactive iodine and cesium, and bee products like pollen and honey were used as markers to monitor the extent of radiological pollution.[12] Although the accident occurred many years ago, some locals still tend to avoid honey from the Chernobyl region because they believe that some of the land (and therefore the plants and products from these plants) in this area remains radioactive.

In Canada, the United States, the United Kingdom, and Italy honey-bees have been used to monitor environmental pollution, because accumu-lations of certain heavy metals and other substances can be measured in pollen, honey, and other hive products, as well as in the bees themselves.

Most of the honey that's sold in supermarkets today is imported in bulk from one or more countries. It is then blended and packaged into plastic or glass containers for sale. The consumer has no idea where the honey actually comes from aside from a label indicating the country (or countries) of origin. This is why a growing number of savvy consumers only buy honey from sources they know and trust, such as individual api-aries, local farm stands, or from distributors that have been awarded a "Certified Organic" label from a reputable organization.

3

SACRED BEE,
SACRED HONEY

Our treasure lies in the beehive of our knowledge. We are
perpetually on the way thither, being by nature winged
insects and honey gatherers of the mind.

FRIEDRICH NIETZSCHE

Rudolf Steiner (1861–1925), the founder of anthroposophy and developer of Waldorf education and biodynamic agriculture, in 1923 gave a series of lectures entirely devoted to bees, beekeeping, and honey. Steiner strongly believed that life in the beehive possessed an extraordinary wisdom and that both bees and honey were vitally connected to our experience of health, culture, and the cosmos.

Unlike humans, who are believed to possess an individual mind and soul, Steiner taught that honeybees, like other insects, are part of a group soul that stands behind and guides their evolution. And by virtue of the bee's connection to flowers and sky, he believed that they serve as an important—and sacred—link between humanity and the heavenly realms. This is one reason why he wrote: "You need to study the life of bees from the standpoint of the soul."[1]

As a prolific provider of honey and other important products, the honey-bee is perhaps humanity's oldest ally. And because our human ancestors viewed the production of honey as a magical alchemical process known only to the bees, they considered both the honeybee and honey as sacred gifts from heaven. Honey was an important offering to the gods in many parts of the ancient world, and both honey and bees have been celebrated in myths and legends in many of the world's cultures. Bees have also been seen as wisdom keepers who teach humanity about the essential virtues of harmony, cooperation, thrift, selflessness, and productivity. As "power animals," bees have long represented many qualities—like fertility, bravery, strength, and innate wisdom—that humans wish to acquire for themselves.

A Distinguished Ancestry

Although the life span of the average worker bee is only two to three months long, the modern honeybee can trace its ancestry back to the Middle Eocene period of the Cenozoic era. A fossilized bee (*Eckfeldapis electrapoides*) was found in Germany that was carbon dated to fifty million years ago, while a fossil of a stingless bee (*Trigona prisca*) found in the state of New Jersey dates from approximately the same time. Humans have been eating honey for the past few million years, and records of human exploitation of bees date back to approximately ten thousand years.

The Arrival of *Apis mellifera*

Flowers first appeared on Earth between 100 and 150 million years ago, and bees eventually joined in their evolutionary process. Solitary bees appeared twenty-five million years ago, and they became social insects about ten to twenty million years ago. The first humans began to evolve much later.

Apis mellifera (literally "bee bringing honey") is the honeybee we know today. Making its evolutionary debut around five million years ago, its name shows that at first humans thought that bees carried honey from the flowers to the hive. The honeybee is believed to have originated in Southeast Asia and eventually extended its distribution into temperate Asia and Europe.

Technically known as the western honeybee, *Apis mellifera* is now found nearly everywhere on Earth, with the exception of the polar regions of the world. Other species that form part of the *Apis* genus have grown to inhabit much of the planet as well: the eastern honeybee (*Apis cerana*), the giant honeybee (*Apis dorsata*), and the dwarf honeybee (*Apis florea*). Only the first two have been domesticated by humans and managed in constructed hives.

The First Honey Hunters

The desire for sweetness is said to be innate in humans, and our earliest ancestors probably developed a taste for honey when they learned how to walk upright. The first honey hunters or honey gatherers are believed to have lived in what is now eastern Spain, as evidenced by a Paleolithic cave painting from Bicorp that is ten thousand years old. The painting depicts two figures standing on a rope ladder, climbing the face of a cliff. The arm of the figure standing at the top is thrust inside a bees' nest, while his other hand grasps a basket in the hope of collecting the honey. A swarm of bees hover angrily around his head. A similar painting that dates between 4500 and 4000 BCE was found in Altamira in northern Spain. Other ancient rock paintings in Spain show one or more men perched precariously on a long, rickety ladder and taking honey from a bees nest high in a tree.

Spain wasn't the only place where humans looked for honey. The largest number of rock paintings depicting honey hunting is found throughout Africa, including present-day Algeria, Lesotho, Libya, Malawi, Morocco, Namibia, South Africa, Tanzania, Tunisia, the western Sahara, and Zimbabwe. Several of the most impressive paintings depicting honeycomb patterns were found in Namibia, while catenary curve patterns (indicating a bees' nest) were most commonly found in South Africa.

Bee hunting continues to this day in many parts of Africa. The !Kung people of southern Africa are said to claim no personal possessions except for their treasured bees' nests. Honey is considered sacred among many African peoples, including the Thonga tribe of southern Africa. According to the Swiss anthropologist Henri A. Junod: "The honey of the wild black bee, which is used by the Bathonga for purposes of divination in magical horns, is obtained by digging out the nests, which are two to three feet underground. Although anyone may eat the honey, the nests can be found only by members of certain families."[2]

Honey in History: The First Beekeepers

The first domesticated hives were believed to have consisted of a bee colony located in part of a hollow log; the wood surrounding the hive was trimmed and transported to the bee hunter's home. It is said that some African peoples continue to raise bees in this way.[3]

Ancient Egypt

Paintings at Çatal Hüyük in Anatolia (in present-day Turkey) dating from around 7000 BCE have been interpreted to depict honeycombs and bees foraging on flowers. However, the first clear evidence of beekeeping is paintings on the walls of the sun temple of Neuserre in ancient Egypt that date from 2400 BCE. According to Eva Crane in her classic text *The Archeology of Beekeeping*:

> These scenes are sufficiently similar to show that in 2400 BC beekeeping was already a well-developed craft, and that it did not change very much in the next 1800 years. We know nothing of its earlier history or chronology. Peasant beekeepers in Egypt today use hives and methods that are fairly similar to those shown in the Ancient Egyptian scenes. There has, in fact, been relatively little change even in 4400 years.[4]

Both bees and honey were considered sacred in ancient Egypt, and honey featured prominently in religious ceremonies, including offerings to the dead. In about 1200 BCE, King Ramses III offered the gods of the Nile tens of thousands of jars filled with honey, estimated to weigh about fifteen tons.

In addition to its use in religious ceremony, the ancient Egyptians considered honey a rare and highly desirable food. They included honey in marriage dowries, and honey was given to high-ranking officials as part of their government rations. Evidence shows that the ancient Egyptians could not get enough of the stuff: they not only produced their own honey but imported it as well.

Assyria, Sumeria, and Babylonia

Both bees and their honey were considered sacred in ancient Assyria, Sumeria, and Babylonia, three cultures that flourished in Mesopotamia, where evidence shows that bees thrived in the lower Euphrates Valley. Honey played an important role in many Assyrian religious rites, and beeswax was used to cast sacred images in bronze, known as *cire perdu,* or the lost wax process. Through this process, which is still done today, anything that can be modeled in wax can be faithfully transmuted into metal, such as fine jewelry and sculpture.

Honey was also used to help consecrate temples, such as the one constructed to honor the god Ningirsu (a Sumero-Babylonian god of rain, irrigation, and fertility) by Gudea, the ruler of Lagash in about 2450 BCE. According to Hilda M. Ransome writing in her classic *The Sacred Bee:* "Honey was poured over thresholds and stones bearing commemorative offerings, and honey and wine were poured over bolts which were to be used in some sacred buildings. Temples were erected on ground which had been consecrated by libations of wine, oil, and honey."[5]

The Assyrians and Babylonians also used honey as an offering when invoking the protection of deities like Ishtar (the goddess of fertility, sexual love, and war) and Marduk (god of water, vegetation, and white magic) against the evils of black magic and witchcraft. They also used honey to help preserve the bodies of the dead.

China

The ancient Chinese first recorded the use of honey at about the same time as the Mesopotamians. It was referred to in writings dating back to 2000 BCE during the Xia dynasty and, more frequently—especially as both food and medicine—during the Southern and Northern Dynasties that reached their highest point around 500 CE. During the Yin dynasty (1523–1028 BCE), the earliest pictographs for honey appear in an inscription on bones. Emperor Trou Yu, who believed bees to be auspicious, had them added to his official flag.

As in Egypt, honey rations were given to high Chinese government functionaries. During the Han dynasty, Emperor Kwan gave seventy-three kilograms of honey to a friend as a gift, while upon retirement, one official was granted a quart of honey each month, amounting to nineteen kilograms a year.[6]

The bee itself has been a sacred image in Chinese culture for at least six thousand years, as evidenced by carvings dating back to the Hongshan culture in northeastern China, which flourished between 4700 and 2900 BCE. Today, Chinese collectors prize small stone carvings of bees based on ancient Hongshan designs—like the jade amulet seen in figure 3.1.

India

Nearly a dozen prehistoric rock paintings of bees and their hives have been found in central India, especially of *Apis dorsata,* the giant honeybee that builds a very large single cone for a nest that hangs down from a tall tree or rock ledge.

Text references to bees and honey first appeared in 1400 BCE in ancient Indian spiritual literature, with eight different types of honey

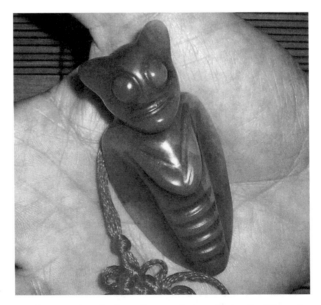

Figure 3.1. Jade Bee Amulet based on a design from the Hongshan culture, northeastern China. Photograph by Nathaniel Altman.

having been linked to specific plants. A sacred group of texts known as the Vedas dating from 1000 BCE praised both the health and spiritual benefits of honey, with instructions that it should be eaten by all human beings and especially by students of religion and philosophy.

The early Indians believed in the inherent purity of honey, and honey was referred to in the Rig-Veda—an ancient Indian sacred collection of Vedic Sanskrit hymns dedicated to the gods—as having divine origin; the early Hindus also believed honey to be food of the gods. Whenever honey was removed from the hive, the person held a purple datura plant (*Datura metel*) that was sacred to Lord Vishnu in his or her hand. In Hindu mythology, Lord Vishnu was often represented as a bee on a lotus leaf, while Lord Krishna has a blue bee on his forehead.

Honey also played a role in early Hindu marriage ceremonies, because it was believed to drive away evil spirits and help assure a harmonious married life. Among the Deccan Hindus honey and curds make up a traditional food given to the groom when he first visits the home of his prospective bride. In some parts of Bengal the bride has certain parts of her body anointed with honey, a custom that also was part of the Roma (gypsy) tradition in the Balkan Peninsula.

We'll see in chapter 4 that honey has long been an integral part of ayurvedic medicine, an ancient system of health care that originated in the Indian subcontinent more than five thousand years ago. Still practiced by thousands of practitioners in India and other parts of the world, ayurveda remains one of the most popular forms of natural health care on the planet today.

Greece

The Ancient Greeks were believed to have learned apiculture from the Egyptians, although Dionysus—the god of both wine and inspired madness—was said to have made the first hives and to have shown his people how to gather honey. In Greece both bees and honey were sacred, and honey was believed to elevate human consciousness: the melodies of poets were said to be inspired by "honey-dropping founts in certain gardens and glades of the Muses."[7]

The Greeks believed that honey came from the heavens. In chapter

12 of book 11 of his huge encyclopedia *Natural History,* the author and natural philosopher Pliny the Elder (23–79 CE) wrote:

> This substance is engendered from the air . . . at early dawn the leaves of the trees are found covered with a kind of honey-like dew. . . . Whether a saliva emanating from the stars, or a juice exuding from the air while purifying itself, would that it had been, when it comes to us, pure, limpid, and genuine, as it was, when first it took its downward descent.[8]

In Greek mythology, honey was fed to the infant Zeus, who later became the god of the sky and thunder, as well as king of the gods. According to legend, the nymph Melissa (meaning honeybee) cared for Zeus while he was being hidden from his father, Cronos. She fed Zeus a diet of honey that she stole from the hives. When discovered, Cronos punished Melissa by turning her into a worm. Zeus knew that she had protected him and kept him alive, so he eventually transformed Melissa into a queen bee.

Like the Assyrians, the ancient Greeks knew that honey could be used to preserve the bodies of the dead. It was recorded that on his death-bed Alexander the Great commanded that his body should be placed "in white honey which had not been melted" and returned to his homeland in a preserved state.

The great mathematician Pythagoras is said to have lived largely on bread and honey for years. Plato, one of the most important philosophers in Greek antiquity, probably remembered his elder's example when he taught that honey is an important part of a moderate and healthy diet. Hesiod (800 BCE), Aristophanes (450–388 BCE), and Varro (116–27 BCE) all spoke about the cultivation of bees, and honey from Attica was considered (and, some argue, still is) the best honey to be found in Greece.

Honey in the Holy Land
The early Hebrews and the Essenes—a Jewish religious group that flourished from the second century BCE to the first century CE—valued wild

honey as one of the finest of foods; they also considered honey a symbol of both abundance and heavenly grace.

The Hebrew Scriptures contain many references to honey. In Exodus 3:8, while addressing Moses from the burning bush, Yahweh announces his plan to bring the Israelites out of Egypt to a "land flowing with milk and honey."

> And I am come down to deliver them out of the hand of the Egyptians, and to bring them up out of that land unto a good land and a spacious land, unto a land flowing with milk and honey; unto the place of the Canaanites, and the Hittites, and the Amorites, and the Perizzites, and the Hivites, and the Jebusites.[9]

Other passages of the Holy Bible abound with references to honey. The Song of Solomon mentions both honey and honeycomb in connection with the bridegroom (5:1) and the bride (4:11), and the Book of Proverbs (16:24) makes allusions to friendly words as "honeycombs." In Genesis 43:11, Jacob sends honey as a gift to Joseph, the powerful governor of Egypt, while in 1 Kings 14:3, Jeroboam asked his wife to bring a gift of honey to the prophet Ahijah, entreating him to heal their sick son. This may be one of the first biblical references to honey as medicine. Honey was valued as a remedy for the eyes in early Israel, and Ahijah suffered from blindness.

Although some early Jews forbade the eating of honey because the bee belonged to a class of "unclean" insects, some rabbis permitted its use because they argued (erroneously) that honey is not the product of the bee, but that honey is merely stored in its body. Today many Jewish families dip bread in honey during the period between Rosh Hashana to Hoshana Rabba, symbolizing the wish for a "good and sweet" New Year. During the Middle Ages a child would write the sacred letters of the Hebrew alphabet on a slate, and the letters would be covered with a thin layer of honey. The young scholar would be encouraged to lick the honey-covered letters off the slate, so that the words of the scriptures might be "as sweet as honey."[10]

Among early Christians, honey had a deep and mysterious meaning. It was served to the newly christened as a symbol of renovation and spiritual perfection. To this day, Russian Christians serve honey on both Christmas Eve—the greatest Christian holiday—and at funeral banquets to help the departed experience spiritual transformation.

While the early Muslims considered honey an important food and medicine, the bee itself was not viewed as a sacred animal. However, the honeybee was revered for its creativity and hard work and is the only animal that Mohammed said was addressed by Allah himself. In the Sunna, an early book about the traditions of Mohammed, honey was described as existing in heaven, and the Holy Qur'an (Sura 47:17, 18) says that there are rivers of honey in the Paradise promised to those who fear Allah.

The honeybee was one of the few animals honored in an entire book of the Holy Qur'an. Verses 68–70 of Sura 16, which bears the simple title "The Bee," reads:

> And thy Lord taught the bee to build its cells in the hills, on trees and in (men's) habitations; then to eat of all the produce (of the earth), and find with skill the spacious paths of its Lord: There issues from within their bodies a drink of varying colors, wherein is healing for men: Verily in this is a sign for those who give thought.[11]

Honey remains important in the Muslim world today. It is not only used as a traditional medicine, but honey is also a major ingredient of many candies and pastries like baklava and Bint al-sahn (honey cake). Some fine honeys, like the rare and expensive Sidr honey from Southern Yemen, are considered among the finest gifts a person can either bestow or receive.

Honey in the Middle Ages

During the Middle Ages in Europe, honey was used as a sweetener, a medicine, and a preservative. Confectioners also utilized it to mix with fruits, nuts, herbs, and spices. In ancient Gaul and early England, the flavor of poor-quality wine was concealed by the addition of honey and spices, a product known today as mulled wine.

Honey was also a major ingredient in mead, also known as "honey wine," a popular alcoholic drink enjoyed throughout the British Isles and northern Europe. Made with honey, yeast, and water, mead was made by fermenting the final washings of honey from the comb in a solution containing yeast and water.

Although almost unknown today, mead was highly valued until as late as the seventeenth century. It was even the subject of myth and legend. In Valhalla, the heaven of Viking warriors, it was said that the Valkyries gave mead to the newcomers. Newly wedded couples were given full honeycombs for a moon's worth of mead. The Celts thought that bees had a secret wisdom that came from the Otherworlds and believed that a river of mead flowed through heaven.

Finnish folklore abounds with references to bees and honey. In the Kalavala, the epic poem of the Finns, the bee is implored to fly over the moon, sun, and stars into the dwelling of the Creator and to carry health and honey to the righteous. In early Finland honey was often used in ointments, as a drink, and as an additive to beer. It was also a popular ingredient for sweetening cakes, including those offered to the forest gods to provide abundant game to the hunter.

Bees and Honey in the New World

Other groups of bees make honey as well. Unlike the *Apis,* the *Meliponini* do not have a stinger. They are native to the Americas and Australia as well as Asia and Africa. The late Eva Crane, perhaps the world's foremost expert on bees, reported that it was their honey that Christopher Columbus referred to when he returned to Spain after his first voyage to America.[12]

The bee was treasured by the early Mexicans, who raised them in boxes made out of straw or wood and in hollowed-out logs. They used the honey primarily as food. As in ancient Sumeria and Babylonia, beeswax was utilized in molds to fashion gold jewelry, religious figurines, and other sacred implements through the lost wax process.

Mayan priests considered the honeybee a sacred being, and the powerful Bee God—known as Ah Muzen Kab—is still worshipped by traditional Mayans today. In times past, sacred bees were raised in a designated building from which honey was taken for use in religious ritual only. The Mayans also made special loaves of honey bread to use as an offering to the gods.

The *Chilam Balam of Chumayel,* a classic in Mayan literature consisting of the memories of the pre-Columbian Maya of the Yucatan, refers to the Bee God as one of the four cardinal directions: "The red flint is the stone of the red Ah Muzen Kab, one who holds up the [eastern] sky who also serves as the Bee God."[13] In the Mexican highlands, bees were also considered sacred and were connected to the gods of the rains, flowers, and happiness.

The early Mayans celebrated the sacred bee in the Codex Tro-Cortesiano, one of the three ancient Mayan codices. Both Ah Muzen Kab and the sacred bee are represented in several pictographs, including those reproduced in figure 3.2.

The Arrival of *Apis mellifera* to America

Native bees populated vast forested areas of North America before the Europeans arrived. Totally undomesticated, they flourished primarily in

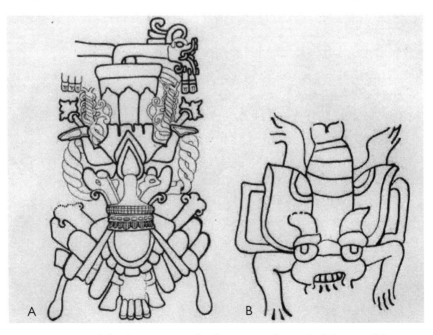

*Figure 3.2. (A) Ah Muzen Kab, the Mayan bee god. (B) Sacred bee.
Reprinted from Ralph M. Roys,* The Book of Chilam Balam
of Chumayal *(Washington: Carnegie Institution, 1933).*

rotting tree trunks, cavities found in cliffs, and holes in the ground.

The first beehive containing *Apis mellifera* was brought to the Virginia colony in North America in 1622, with additional bees arriving in New England during the 1630s.

In her delightful book *Sweetness and Light: The Mysterious History of the Honeybee,* Hattie Ellis writes that the town of Newbury, Massachusetts, boasted a communal apiary in 1640. Bees were said to thrive in Swedish settlements in Pennsylvania and in the Boston area as well. By the time of the American Revolution, most farms in the thirteen colonies had at least one beehive, and many contained several.

Yet many honeybee colonies did not want to live in hives and decided to make a life of their own. By the early 1800s, the migration of *Apis mellifera* was said to move westward at a rate of six hundred miles every fourteen years.[14]

Members of the Church of Jesus Christ of Latter-day Saints, often colloquially referred to as the Mormons, were the first to bring bee colonies to their new settlements in what is now Utah in 1847. The image of the beehive and the term "Industry" were unofficial symbols of the region. In 1847 the provisional state of Deseret, which was to become Utah, adopted the beehive as its official emblem. The qualities of the beehive (industry, perseverance, thrift, stability, and self-reliance) were virtues respected by the early Mormons. This symbol became part of the Great Seal of the state of Utah when it joined the Union in 1896, as seen in figure 3.3.

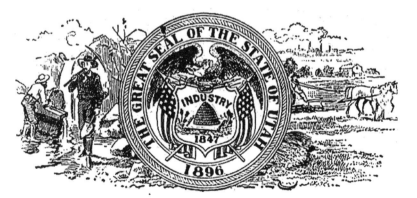

Figure 3.3. The great seal of the state of Utah

Native Americans and Honey

Although Native Americans had collected honey from the nests of wild bees for centuries, they were not familiar with either the honeybee or beekeeping until the Europeans arrived. They were impressed at how the white settlers managed to have an insect work for them as diligently as the honeybee did. Some tribes, including the Cherokee, later practiced bee-keeping themselves, and some developed folklore about the magical powers of the bee. According to the contemporary Native American healer Bobby "Medicine Grizzly Bear" Lake-Thom, the bee is a power animal that can be used for fertility, protection, and love power. He also believes that the bee is a messenger with news about sex when a visitor calls: "If you see a bee fly close by or in your house, then you know what is on the person's mind who came to visit."[15] An outstanding bee mask created by Rupert Scow Jr., a member of the Kwagiulth Nation in British Columbia (part of the Kwakiutl region), is reproduced in figure 3.4.

In his beautiful essay entitled "The Bee-Pastures of California," first published in *The Century Illustrated Monthly Magazine* in 1882, naturalist John Muir observed: "When California was wild, it was one sweet bee-garden throughout its entire length, north and south, and all the way across from the snowy Sierra to the ocean." He called the Great Central

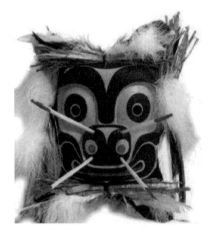

Figure 3.4. Bee Mask by Rupert Scow Jr. Photograph by Sara Wark. Courtesy of Appleton Galleries, Vancouver, BC, © 2007 by Appleton Galleries. All rights reserved.

Plain "one smooth, continuous bed of honey-bloom" during the spring, with a carpet so dense that "your foot would press about a hundred flowers at every step."[16]

Such an environment was perfect for beekeeping, and *Apis mellifera* thrived. The first honeybee colony was brought into Los Angeles County in 1854, three years after the American apiarist L. I. Langworth introduced scientific beekeeping, a system based on the tenets of covered bee space and the movable-frame hive. The original Los Angeles honeybee colony soon multiplied, and by 1876 there were an estimated fifteen thousand to twenty thousand beehives in California, with some bee ranches containing more than one thousand hives. Eventually California became one of the largest honey-producing states in the country and is home to a variety of both common and exotic honeys, including fireweed, tanbark, tarweed, lotus blossom, echinacea, meadow foam, and blue curl. An illustration of a rustic bee ranch from Muir's article appears in figure 3.5.

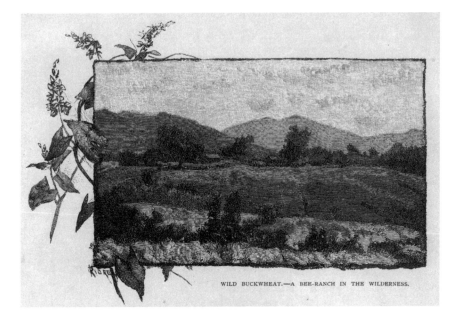

WILD BUCKWHEAT.—A BEE-RANCH IN THE WILDERNESS.

Figure 3.5. "Wild Buckwheat—A Bee-Ranch in the Wilderness."
From John Muir, "The Bee-Pastures of California," 1882.

Australia and New Zealand

Honeybees were first brought to New South Wales in Australia in 1822, where stingless bees had been living for millions of years and their honey collected by the Aborigines for centuries. *Apis mellifera* arrived in the North Island of New Zealand from England in 1839 and soon began to thrive in that beautiful and fertile land. One of the most colorful early promoters of honeybees in New Zealand was William Cotton, an eccentric English cleric. Because bees had not previously existed in New Zealand, he introduced the indigenous Māori to the sweetness of honey and later taught them how to raise bees themselves. Rev. Cotton was also a tireless advocate of humane beekeeping, and he campaigned strenuously against the practice of killing bees when the honey was harvested in the fall. He admonished: "NEVER KILL YOUR BEES . . . every one of you must feel some sorrow when you murder by thousands in the autumn those who have worked hard for you all the summer, and are ready to do so again next year."[17]

The Honeybee Today

As modern science has demystified the sacred *Apis mellifera* and has scientifically explained its activities that used to be viewed as magical, humans have grown to disregard the importance of this amazing animal to the extent that we take the western honeybee (and the honey it produces) completely for granted.

Yet the well-being of *Apis mellifera* remains vital to human survival. In years past farmers whose crops needed cross-pollination rented several honeybee colonies from a local beekeeper every season. When the plants began to bloom, the beekeeper—perhaps with the help of family members or neighbors—would quietly move the bees to a nearby orchard or field, usually at night when all the bees were safely in the hive.

Today agriculture has become big business, and more than 2.5 million honeybee colonies are rented for pollination each year in the United States alone. Instead of being transported short distances at night by sensitive beekeepers, many beehives are loaded onto trucks and transported over large distances throughout the growing season: from almond groves in California, to fields of clover in the Midwest, to blueberry farms in the East, and back again. As we will see in chapter 15, the large-scale commercial interstate shipping of bees is one of the prime suspects behind Colony Collapse Disorder (CCD), a little-understood phenomenon in which worker bees from a beehive or western honeybee colony abruptly disappear.

Although honey has always been an important bee-related product, pollination is where the money is made: literally millions of acres of fruit, vegetable, oilseed, and legumes depend on the honeybee for pollination. While some plants can be pollinated by other insects, numerous crops—including apples, avocados, blueberries, cherries, cranberries, sunflowers, alfalfa, cucumbers, kiwi fruit, melons, and many vegetables—are pollinated mostly by honeybees. The issues of large-scale pollination and Colony Collapse Disorder will be addressed in more detail in the final chapters of this book.

4

HONEY IN MEDICINE

The time has now come for conventional medicine to lift the blinds off this "traditional remedy" and give it its due recognition.

ALIMUDDIN ZUMLA, M.D., AND A. LULAT, M.D.,
WRITING ABOUT HONEY IN THE
JOURNAL OF THE ROYAL SOCIETY OF MEDICINE

On July 23, 2007, Derma Sciences, an American distributor of medical supplies, announced approval by the U.S. Food and Drug Administration (FDA) to sell its range of Medihoney brand wound dressings produced by Comvita, a New Zealand company. Although honey-based wound dressings have been available in New Zealand, Australia, the United Kingdom, and other European countries for at least a decade, they had never been licensed for sale in the United States, purportedly the most medically advanced country in the world.

While still considered a new product by the majority of American health care practitioners, honey dressings—like other honey-based medicines—have been around for more than five thousand years. Honey was an ingredient in more than half of the medicinal compounds and cures developed by early Egyptian physicians. Honey has also played an important role in both traditional Chinese medicine and in ayurveda, a natural healing system developed in India thousands of years ago.

Egypt

The Edwin Smith Surgical Papyrus, a unique Egyptian surgical treatise dating from the seventeenth century BCE (figure 4.1), is considered the most ancient medical text of humankind. Named in honor of the British Egyptologist who first purchased the papyrus in Luxor in 1862, it is now preserved in the archives at the New York Academy of Medicine. The document not only describes forty-eight cases of breaks, wounds, and sprains in detail but also outlines a recommended treatment for each.

Many entries include medical advice for healing skin gashes, ulcers, and other open wounds, including instructions for treating a gaping wound of the temple that penetrates to the bone with honey: "[Thou] shouldst bind [fresh meat upon it the first day; thou shouldst apply for him two strips of linen, and treat afterward with grease, honey, (and) lint]

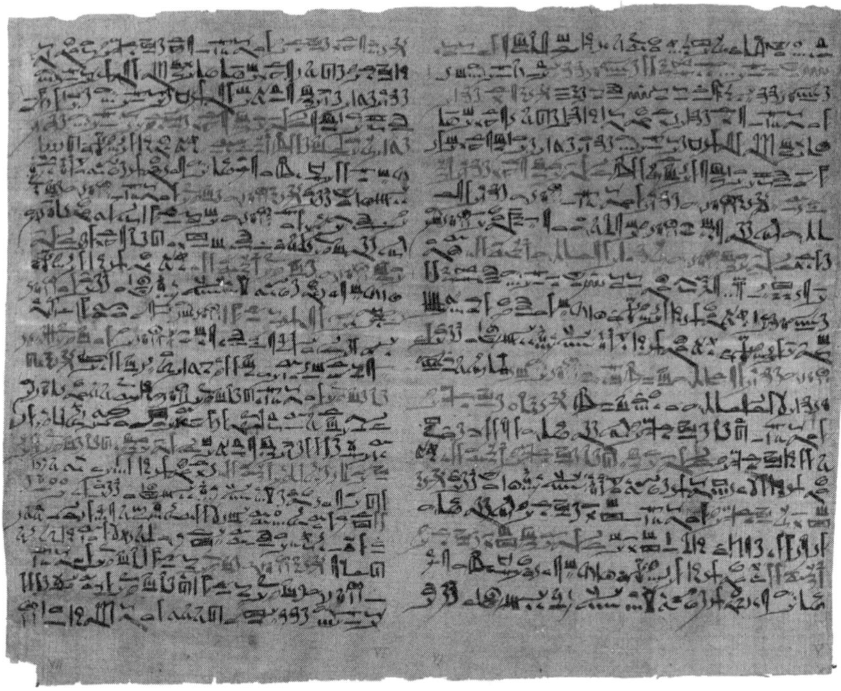

Figure 4.1. Plates 6 and 7 of the Edwin Smith Papyrus

every day until he recovers."[1] Honey—often mixed with lint as a binder—is the standard antiseptic of *The Edwin Smith Surgical Papyrus*. In fact, of the nine hundred remedies mentioned in this renowned medical text, approximately five hundred call for the use of honey. Not only was honey used as an antiseptic dressing, but it was also a major ingredient in healing unguents and salves.

Honey also appears frequently in the formulae of the Ebers Papyrus (ca. 1550 BCE), which mentions 147 external-use prescriptions containing honey. In the Assyrian Empire of northern Mesopotamia, whose "First Golden Age" lasted between 2400 BCE to 612 BCE, honey-based medicines were used to treat problems of both the eyes and ears.

Greece

I mentioned earlier that the Greeks believed that honey was an important part of a healthy diet. Pythagoras (who lived between 580 and 572 BCE to between 500 and 490 BCE) attributed his long life to eating honey regularly. Many of his followers adopted his practice. Aristoxenus (ca. 350 BCE), a disciple of Aristotle, claimed that those who eat honey for breakfast will be free from disease for life, while Aristotle himself wrote in book 9, chapter 40 of his *Historia Animalium* that "white honey . . . is good as a salve for sore eyes and wounds."[2]

One of the best-known Greek stories about healing honey concerns the philosopher Democritus, who wanted to die in his 110th year. He ate less and less food each day. But an important festival approached and the women in his household persuaded him not to die during the holiday. According to a translation of the ancient Greek text *Deipnosophistae II:* ". . . He was persuaded and ordered a vessel full of honey to be set near him, and in this way he lived for many days with no other support than the honey; and then some days afterwards when the honey had been taken away, he died."[3]

Although honey was not a specific part of Hippocratic medicine, Hippocrates listed several virtues of honey: "It causes heat, cleans sores and ulcers, softens hard ulcers of the lips, heals carbuncles and running sores."[4]

Dioscorides of Anazarbus was a Greek physician born in southeast

Asia Minor in the Roman Empire in the first few decades CE. During his lifetime, Dioscorides traveled extensively seeking medicinal substances from all over the Greek and Roman world. In his famous work known in Latin as *De materia medica,* he wrote of honey being "good for sunburn and spots on the face." He also taught that "honey heals inflammation of the throat and tonsils, and cures coughs" and even "mollifies the prepuce so that it can be pulled back over the penis."[5]

Rome

In ancient Rome, the philosopher and naturalist Pliny the Elder (23–79 CE) wrote that Roman doctors using honey mixed with aloe cured bruises, burns, and abrasions. In his book *Naturalis Historia* he gave a long list of other bodily disorders for which he believed honey to be an effective remedy.

> As to honey itself, it is of so peculiar a nature, that it prevents putrefaction from supervening, by reason of its sweetness solely, and not any inherent acridity, its natural properties being altogether different from those of salt. It is employed with the greatest success for affections of the throat and tonsils, for quinsy and all ailments of the mouth, as also in fever, when the tongue is parched. Decoctions of it are used also for peri-pneumony and pleurisy, for wounds inflicted by serpents, and for the poison of fungi. For paralysis, it is prescribed in honeyed wine, though that liquor also has its own peculiar virtues. Honey is used with rose-oil, as an injection for the ears; it has the effect also of exterminating nits and foul vermin of the head. It is the best plan always to skim it before using it.[6]

As in Assyria, Roman physicians considered honey to be an effective remedy for ear infections. Galen (130–201 CE) wrote that warm honey "wonderfully helps exulcerated ears, especially if they cast forth ill flavors." The medical writer Marcellus Empiricus wrote that an equal amount of honey, butter, and rose oil "warms, helps the pain of the ears, dullness of the sight and white spots in the eyes."[7]

Ancient Israel

The Talmud, a record of rabbinical discussions pertaining to Jewish law, ethics, customs, and history, mentions the use of honey to treat eye diseases. Yoma 83b reads: "If one is seized with a ravenous hunger, he is given to eat honey, for honey enlightens the eyes of men." First Samuel 14:27 refers to Jonathan, the son of King Saul, who ate honey and "his eyes became bright."[8]

India

In Ancient India honey became an important part of ayurvedic medicine wherein physicians believed it helped other ingredients in a healing formula work more strongly. A honey-based paste was used after surgery. Susruta, an early ayurvedic surgeon who lived around 1400 BCE, treated infected wounds with a paste made of honey and clarified butter (ghee) enriched with barley and herbs. Lotus honey is still considered to be an effective remedy for eye diseases.

In ayurvedic medicine, honey possesses a variety of medicinal properties and is classified as "heavy" (*guru guna*), "dry" (*ruksha*), or "cold" (*sheeta*). According to the text *Honey and Its Ayurvedic Approach,* practitioners have classified eight distinct types of medicinal honey depending on the type of bee that collects it.

1. Large, bluish honeybees collect makshika honey. Ayurvedic practitioners consider it "very light and dry natured" and use it to treat both vata kapha diseases and kapha diseases like jaundice, hemorrhoids, coughs, tuberculosis, and eye diseases. Considered the finest of all honey types, makshika is said to contain immense medicinal properties.

2. Pouttika honey is collected by small bees that live in the hollows of old trees. This type of honey increases vata dosha (a type of energy that governs all movement) and creates a burning sensation in the chest. It is used to treat diabetes and to reduce the size of tumors.

3. Bhramara honey is collected by another type of small bee and is

both very sticky and transparent white in color. Ayurvedic practitioners use it to cure urinary tract disorders, digestive problems, and blood-related diseases.

4. Kshoudra is a honey collected by medium-size brown honeybees. Considered light and cold in nature, it dissolves kapha dosha, which governs the structural integrity of the body. It is similar to makshika honey in healing properties and is especially used to treat diabetes.

5. Collected by a brown and yellow bee that builds honeycombs in Himalayan forests, chatra honey is called "heavy and cold." It is used to treat symptoms of gout, indigestion, and worms. Ayurvedic doctors also consider it a good honey for overall nourishment.

6. Arghya honey is made by a yellow bee. It is primarily used to treat eye problems and is recommended for general nourishment.

7. Auddalaka honey is made by a small brown bee that lives in anthills. An astringent, auddalaka honey is used to treat skin diseases; it is also taken internally to improve voice modulation.

8. Dala honey is considered "dry" and is good for digestion. Ayurvedic doctors prescribe this honey to reduce vomiting and treat diabetes.[9]

Honey and Its Ayurvedic Approach includes no fewer than 634 ayurvedic remedies that contain honey to treat an incredibly wide range of health problems. They include tuberculosis, bronchitis, fever, celiac disease (sprue), parasites, kidney stones, heart disease, diabetes, asthma, anemia, jaundice, gout, epilepsy, colic, leg stiffness, fainting, mental disease, vomiting, rheumatism, dyspnea (difficulty breathing), edema, obesity, smallpox, chickenpox, alopecia, stomatitis, syphilis, metrorrhagia (irregular uterine bleeding), leprosy, hemorrhoids, and hiccup.

Some ayurvedic recipes are very complex and include a dozen or more ingredients, while others are deceptively simple. For example, to increase hydration in those suffering from diarrhea, a drink made of pomegranate juice and lemon juice mixed with honey is recommended, while honey added to the juice of the fruit of the Palash or Parrot tree (*Butea monosperma*) is indicated for eliminating intestinal worms.[10]

Traditional Chinese Medicine

In ancient China the first mention of honey as a medicine was made during the Xin dynasty by Shen Nang around 2000 BCE. A book on Chinese medicine published during the Qin dynasty around 220 BCE reads: "Those who often take honey can keep fit, honey can cure indigestion, it can be used in medicaments to bind other ingredients together."[11] The famous Ming dynasty physician Li Shizen saw five major medicinal benefits of honey, including relaxation, detoxification, and pain reduction. Honey and warm milk has been a traditional Chinese remedy to treat gastritis and stomach ulcer for centuries, and eating honey has long been a popular treatment for anxiety and insomnia.

Today, honey remains an important part of traditional Chinese healing practice. According to *Fundamentals of Chinese Medicine,* honey contains the following properties that affect the energy channels of the body (meridians) and also treat specific symptoms of injury and illness.

> Balanced; sweet; nontoxic. Enters the lung, spleen and large intestine channels. Supplements the center and moistens the lung; relieves pain and resolves toxin . . . Treats cough due to lung dryness; constipation due to dryness of the intestines; stomach pain; deep-source nasal congestion; mouth sores; scalds and burns.[12]

Traditional Chinese doctors recommend honey either alone or in combination with other healing agents to treat specific health problems. For example, honey is often used in combination with ginseng, dried rehmannia root, poria, and other traditional Chinese herbs to treat dry or lingering cough and to stimulate *qi* (or *chi*), or life force. For colds or abdominal pain, traditional healers suggest using honey combined with peony root, licorice, or cinnamon: this is intended to warm the middle jiao (one of the traditional "three burners" in Chinese medicine and related to the middle of the body) and alleviate pain. Honey is also added to boiling water or used in combination with Chinese angelica root, hemp seed, or other herbs to relieve constipation.

Healing Honey in Islam

I mentioned in the previous chapter that the early Muslims revered bees for their intelligence, industry, and creativity. The Holy Koran devotes an entire chapter to bees and specifically mentions honey as a medicine: "There issues from within their bodies a drink of varying colors, wherein is healing for men."[13]

The prophet Mohammed often spoke about the healing power of honey. According to Ibn Magih, the prophet said, "Honey is a remedy for every illness, and the Koran is a remedy for all illnesses of the mind, therefore I recommend to you both remedies, the Koran and honey."[14] In her book *The Sacred Bee,* Hilda Ransome recounted a story told by the early commentator Al Beidawi about how the prophet Mohammed specifically recommended honey for healing the sick.

> A man went to Mohammed and told him his brother had violent pains in his body, and the prophet told him to give the sick man honey. He did as he was told, but soon came back to say that his brother was no better. Mohammed answered, "Go back and give him more honey, for God speaks the truth, thy brother's body lies." When the honey was taken again, the sick man, thanks to the grace of God, recovered immediately.[15]

In *The World History of Beekeeping and Honey Hunting,* Eva Crane included a translation of a passage by the Muslim physician Ibn el-Beithar, who wrote about honey in his book on herbal medicine, which he wrote near the end of the twelfth century.

> Honey dispels humour (body fluids), relaxes the bowels, is helpful in treating dropsy, preserves flesh and prevents putrefaction, stimulates the appetite, is good against facial tic. Mixed with sesame oil and boiled wine it is used as an emetic when poison had been swallowed. It is the best treatment for gums, and for teeth which it also whitens; it gives good results with tonsillitis; it stimulates coitus; taken with water it cleanses intestinal ulcers and enhances the effect of medication.[16]

Ibn el-Beithar, who lived in what is now Spain, added that heated honey is useful for treating stomach chills, swelling of the intestines, and stomach disorders due to problems of the pituitary gland.[17] Early Muslim physicians also fed honey to their patients as a laxative and also used it to improve blood circulation and to relieve stomach pain. Honey was also fed to children to prevent scurvy and rickets.

Medieval Europe

During the Dark Ages, little was written about the therapeutic uses of honey. Among the few books that mentioned honey was the Saxon herbal *The Leech Book of Bald,* written around 1000 CE. It recommends honey for treating sties, dirty wounds, internal wounds, amputated limbs, and the removal of scabs.[18]

An anonymous surgical treatise written in 1446 included a detailed description of using honey and alum to treat skin ulcers, while the Rev. Charles Butler wrote about honey to clean and disinfect skin wounds and as a mouthwash for ulcers in the seminal bee treatise *The Feminine Monarchie* in 1623.[19]

In Germany, Jos. Roach's *Parnassus medicinalis,* a medical text published in Ulm in 1663, eulogized the healing power of honey in verse.

> *Der Honig treibt den Harn*
> *Und ist zur Lunge gut,*
> *Von Husten, Faulung auch*
> *Es stark bewahren tut.*
>
> *["Honey drives the urine,*
> *is good to the lungs*
> *and is a strong protector*
> *against cough and decay."]*[20]

John Hill published the first English book entirely devoted to honey in 1759. He included several chapters about the medicinal value of honey and how it could be helpful to reduce phlegm and as a cure for tuberculosis, coughs, and hoarseness.

Finland

I mentioned earlier that the epic Finnish poem *The Kalevala* often referred to bees and their magical powers. One story, known as "Lemminkainen's Recovery and Return Home" (Runo xv), recounts the trials of Lemminkainen, a handsome yet reckless young man who journeyed to a village to ask for the hand of the fairest maiden in the land. A jealous cowherd killed the young suitor, cut his body into eight pieces, and threw them into a river. When Lemminkainen's mother heard the news, she brought a magic rake to retrieve her son's body parts from the river. Although she soon managed to piece the body together, her son could neither move nor speak. The mother enlisted the help of a bee to bring her a magical honey-based ointment from heaven. She beseeched:

> *O thou bee, thou bird of honey,*
> *King of all the woodland flowerets,*
> *Go thou forth to seek for honey . . .*
> *From the cup of many a flower,*
> *And the plumes of grasses many,*
> *As an ointment for the patient,*
> *And quite restore the sick one.*[21]

The heroic bee eventually flew past the moon, the sun, and the stars until she arrived at the storeroom of the Almighty to retrieve the heavenly healing substance. The mother anointed her son's body with the magical ointment, and Lemminkainen rose up completely cured.

It should come as no surprise that in Finland honey was an important ingredient in healing ointments for wounds and skin infections. It was also mixed with beer as a drink and was used to sweeten cakes.

Ireland and America

The Irish also believed in the healing power of honey, which has long been a traditional folk remedy. A story that appeared in the *Journal of American Folklore* in 1889 recounted the tale of Mark Flaherty, a young Irishman made ill by an angry warlock who attacked him while he rode in the meadows after sunset. By the morning after the encounter, Flaherty's hair had turned completely white, and he lost so much weight that he became nothing but skin and bones. The story goes:

> One day a beggar came to him and said, "You must go to the bees and fetch so much honey that you can rub yourself all over with it from head to foot. But you must fetch the honey yourself, if anyone does it for you, it won't do you any good. The bees fly to all the flowers, suck the goodness out of them and mix this in their honey. It will cure you, make your hair brown again, and your face fresh and red." The young Irishman followed the beggar's advice and was soon completely cured.[22]

Contemporary Folk Medicine

Honey is used today by traditional healers in Ghana to treat leg ulcers and by Nigerian healers to treat earache. Folk healers in Mali use honey in the topical treatment of measles and in the eyes of measles sufferers to prevent corneal scarring. African folk healers also use honey to treat peptic ulcers.[23]

Some of the finest honey in the world comes from the Wadi Du'an region of Yemen, where it is collected by beekeepers whose ancestors harvested the first honey thousands of years ago. Elderly Yemeni men eat a daily spoonful of wildflower honey to help stay young, while young Yemeni men believe that regular doses will help them father a son. Wildflower honey is also given to new mothers to help them regain their strength after childbirth. The Yemeni people are said to be the highest per capita honey consumers in the world.

In *Honey: The Gourmet Medicine*, Joe Traynor recounts the story of a veterinarian who served in the Bulgarian army as an officer during the Second Balkan War of 1913. His beleaguered platoon had come across a small amount of honey in an abandoned farmhouse. There was not enough honey to use as food for the soldiers, but the officer decided to apply it to the wounds of a few of his men, as medicine was scarce. The officer recorded the case of one soldier, whose infected foot had not responded to medication.

War invalid S., aged 25, had a big scar on the back of his right foot. In the center of the scar was an ulcer three by three centimeters with a deep glossy, grayish bottom and necrotic thickened edges. The patient said the wound had been in this state for three months. . . . Twenty days after the honey ointment was applied the ulcer healed.[24]

Many folk healers still use honey to treat skin ulcers, cuts, and a wide variety of wounds. In rural Ghana honey is a popular treatment for infected leg ulcers, whereas European and American healers use honey either by itself or combined with other ingredients to treat both minor and serious wounds. In his classic *The Nature Doctor,* first published in 1952, the Swiss naturopath Alfred Vogel recommended mixing a teaspoon of honey with twenty to thirty drops of tincture of echinacea for healing minor scrapes, wounds, and cuts. He also suggested the following combination:

For wounds that are refusing to heal properly, mix some honey with 10 per cent horseradish; the horseradish can be finely grated, or use the fresh juice or tincture. Apply this reliable natural remedy to the affected part, and you will be surprised at the good result.[25]

In rural Nigeria traditional healers have long utilized "jungle honey," a rare honey collected from timber and blossom by honeybees living in tropical forests. The healers not only use jungle honey to heal wounds, burns, and skin irritation but also to treat colds and help patients maintain overall wellness.[26]

Honey has also been an important element among practitioners of traditional Russian folk medicine. In many countries that were once part of the former Soviet Union, many physicians receive instruction in both herbal medicine and traditional medicine in medical school.

As befitting such a large geographic area, there are dozens of different types of honey in the former Soviet Union, and many individual honeys have been found to have specific healing properties.

- In addition to being used as an antiseptic to treat wounds and skin infections, meadow honey, for example, is believed to regulate intestinal and liver function.
- May honey, which is made from the first spring flowers, has strongly marked fever-reducing, painkilling, and antibacterial effects. It is widely used to treat cough, headache, fatigue, and fever. May honey is also useful to strengthen hair.
- Mineral-rich buckwheat honey is used both alone and with herbal preparations to lower blood pressure and to relieve symptoms of rheumatism, scarlet fever, measles, and spotted fever. It is also taken internally to prevent and treat blood vessels after radiotherapy, and it is prescribed to patients suffering from radiation sickness.

The Jumla people of western Nepal also use honey in traditional medicine, both by itself and as an ingredient in herbal preparations. In her presentation about apitherapy at an International Bee Research Association (IBRA) Conference in Thailand in March 2000, apiculturist Naomi M. Saville reported:

> The importance of unheated honey as a medicine is well known to the Jumla people. Traditionally raw unheated honey combined with *Picrorhiza scrophulariaefolia* (locally known as katuko or kutki) cured coughs. It is well known as a treatment for heartburn, gastric disorders, stomach ulcers, chapped skin, spots and boils, burns, effects of altitude (when combined with buckwheat flour), snake bites, poisoning, and for many other problems.[27]

Professor Eraldo Medeiros Costa-Neto of the Feira de Santana State University in Brazil reports that different types of honey is used as medicine to treat specific illnesses by native and traditional peoples in the state of Bahia in northeastern Brazil. Among the Pankarare people, for example, honeys from different species of stingless bee are used to treat diabetes, bronchitis, oral mycosis, colds, sore throat, and even impotence. The Pankarare also use honey externally to treat bites by poisonous snakes and rabid dogs.[28]

In the Afro-Brazilian Remanso community living in the Chapada Diamantina National Park, honey from various types of bees is used to treat several common health problems. Honey from *Apis mellifera* (known locally as *oropa*) and the stingless bee *Melipona scutellaris* (*urucu*) is eaten to relieve cough. Honey from another stingless bee, *Scaptotrigona* sp. (*jitai*), is eaten to treat the flu.[29]

Costa-Neto also reported that honey from two other stingless Melipona bees is consumed as general fortifiers by the traditional people in Tanquinho. They also eat the honey of the *Tetragonisca* sp. (another stingless bee) to treat cataracts, glaucoma, and cough.[30]

Yet the use of honey as medicine is no longer limited to ancient cultures and traditional folk healers. In the following chapters we'll explore why honey is becoming recognized as a powerful healing agent and how it is being used in modern medicine.

PART II

Honey as Healer

5

HOW DOES HONEY HEAL?

Honey seems especially indicated when wounds become infected or fail to close or heal. It is probably even more indicated on the wounds left by laparoscopic surgery to remove cancer.

FAISAL RAUF KHAN, M.D., NATIONAL
HEALTH SERVICE TRUST, UNITED KINGDOM

On the morning of October 26, 2007, readers of the *New York Post* woke up to the screaming headline: "SUPERBUG KILLS NYC KID." The story related how a twelve-year-old Brooklyn schoolboy, who was diagnosed with a MRSA infection several weeks before, died in the hospital after antibiotics could not save him.[1]

Several months earlier, a headline in the *Manchester Evening News* in England asked, "Could This Bee How We Defeat Superbug?" The article reported how honey can destroy drug-resistant bacteria like MRSA. It added that manuka honey is used in New Zealand's largest hospital to control MRSA and other bacterial infections.[2]

These contrasting articles point out a tragic fact: while honey is prized for its antibacterial properties in countries like New Zealand and England, it remains almost completely ignored in the United States.

Honey and Bacteria: The Scientific Research

Even though both early physicians and practitioners of folk medicine were amazed at honey's ability to heal, they never recognized its antibacterial properties—honey was simply known to be an effective remedy. This should not be surprising: it is only since the latter part of the nineteenth century that doctors found out that many ailments are the result of infection by microorganisms such as bacteria, fungi, and viruses.

The scientific community has known about honey's antibacterial properties for more than a century, when the Dutch scientist Van Ketel first reported his findings in 1882. Unfortunately, the reasons why honey is such a powerful therapeutic agent haven't been seriously investigated until only recently. Why is this?

A major reason for this lack of interest is that honey is essentially a non-patentable substance that is very inexpensive to produce and use. Most people can simply run to the local farmers' market or natural food store for a jar of therapeutic honey.

While small companies like New Zealand–based Comvita are making money with their honey-based antiseptics and bandages, large pharmaceutical companies—which produce about three-quarters of the approximately $300 billion worth of medications sold in the United States each year—prefer to develop medications that will bring more substantial profits than simple honey creams or dressings. They generally see little financial incentive to incorporate honey-related products into traditional medical practice.

Most of the research money given to medical schools and other research facilities to develop new medications comes from the same pharmaceutical companies. Researchers generally do not receive funding to investigate something as simple and inexpensive as honey. Those who have done research in this field usually receive minimal funding from the government. Some obtain modest grants from organizations like the National Honey Board, an American group representing the honey industry.

In the next few chapters, we'll see how honey is being used to treat a broad spectrum of specific health problems. When compared to antibiotics, honey is extremely cheap. In addition, many people are able to treat themselves with honey at home, either with or without medical supervision. For these reasons, honey poses a threat to the pharmaceutical industry, hospitals, and physicians accustomed to providing expensive drugs, complex medical procedures, and costly hospital stays for many of the ailments that honey can treat at a fraction of the cost.

Because United States government agencies like the FDA and the National Institutes of Health (NIH) are influenced by the pharmaceutical industry and the medical lobby, objective investigation and development of effective protocols regarding therapeutic honey in the United States have been difficult to undertake. This is the main reason why the vast majority of the research presented in this book has been done in other countries like New Zealand, Australia, Canada, and the United Kingdom, where large pharmaceutical companies have less of an impact on national health care policy.

Honey: A Broad-spectrum Killer of Bacteria

During the past dozen years or so, researchers from around the world not only have been discovering how honey heals but also have identified more than 250 clinical strains of bacteria honey can kill. These include *Alcaligenes faecalis, Citrobacter freundii, Escherichia coli, Helicobacter pylori, Enterobacter aerogenes, Salmonella enteridis, Pseudomonas aeruginosa, Acinetobacter calcoaceticus, Klebsiella pneumoniae,* and vancomycin-resistant enterococci (VRE). Perhaps most impressive is the finding that most raw honeys can effectively kill MRSA, the much-feared "superbug" that was responsible for an estimated 94,000 life-threatening infections and 18,650 deaths in 2005.[3]

MRSA is a subgroup (making up about 40 percent) of the common *Staph. aureus* bacterium that is resistant to antibiotics, including penicillin and related drugs. Though MRSA is only one of several bacteria that have become resistant to most antibiotics, it accounts for the majority of infections today. This bacterium thrives in a hospital setting, which is where most people become infected. A patient with a hospital-acquired MRSA infection is about seven times more likely to die than a patient who is not infected.

Species of Bacteria and Their Related Diseases Found to Be Sensitive to Honey Antibacterial Activity

Pathogen	Infection Caused
Bacillus anthracis	anthrax
Corynebacterium diphtheriae	diphtheria
Escherichia coli	diarrhea, septicemia, urinary infections, wound infections
Haemophilus influenzae	ear infections, meningitis, respiratory infections, sinusitis
Klebsiella pneumoniae	pneumonia
Listeria monocytogenes	meningitis
Mycobacterium tuberculosis	tuberculosis
Pasteurella multocida	infected animal bites
Proteus species	septicemia, urinary infections, wound infections
Pseudomonas aeruginosa	urinary and wound infections
Salmonella species	diarrhea
Salmonella cholerae-suis	septicemia
Salmonella typhi	typhoid
Salmonella typhimurium	wound infections
Serratia marcescens	septicemia, wound infections
Shigella species	dysentery
Staphylococcus aureus	abscesses, boils, carbuncles, impetigo, wound infections
Streptococcus faecalis	urinary infections
Streptococcus mutans	dental caries
Streptococcus pneumoniae	ear infections, impetigo, puerperal fever, rheumatic fever, scarlet fever, sore throat, wound infections
Vibrio cholerae	cholera

Source: E. W. Nester, et al. *Microbiology,* second edition (New York: Holt, Rinehart and Winston, 1978).

Honey as Bactericide

A growing body of scientific evidence shows that the effectiveness of honey in many of its medical uses is probably due to its antibacterial activity. There are many reports of the bactericidal activity of honey as well as its bacteriostatic activity, which inhibits the growth of bacteria without actually destroying it.

When we review the numerous reports of the antimicrobial activity of honey, we see that a pattern emerges: honey either kills or inhibits the growth of a wide range of bacterial and fungal species, including many that cause serious infections. However, there are ailments that may be treated with honey that have not yet had the infectious agents tested for their sensitivity to honey's antimicrobial activity. Also, there has not been much distinction made in the different types of antimicrobial activity in honey to which the various microbial species are sensitive.

The Problem with Wounds

In normal situations, like a cut finger or a grazed knee, the wound will heal on its own. But sometimes wounds can become infected with bacteria and they don't heal. Bacteria feed on the injured tissue, multiplying in the wound and causing more tissue damage. The wound starts to smell, and pus collects. This pus is made up of dead white blood cells, which are part of the body's effort to kill the bacteria and heal the infection.

Honey helps wounds to heal by killing the infecting bacteria. Honey has four main properties that help it to exterminate bacteria: osmosis, high acidity, hydrogen peroxide activity, and a variety of phytochemicals that are derived both from the honeybees and the plants they visit.

The Power of Osmosis

When honey is applied to a wound, it acts like a dry sponge that soaks up water. This is a process called osmosis. Because of osmosis, the honey draws fluid away from the infected wound. This helps to kill bacteria, because bacteria need liquid in order to grow.

According to Arne Simon, M.D., and colleagues from the University of Bonn, the Institute for Bee Research (Celle, Germany), and the University of Waikato: "Honey works differently from antibiotics, which attack the bacteria's cell wall or inhibit intracellular metabolic pathways. Honey is hygroscopic, meaning it draws moisture out of the environment and thus dehydrates bacteria."[4]

This happens because honey is a saturated (or supersaturated) solution of sugars, with 84 percent of the honey being a mixture of fructose and glucose. The water content in honey is usually only 15–21 percent by weight. The strong interaction of these sugar molecules with water molecules leaves very few of the water molecules available to support the survival—let alone growth—of microorganisms.[5]

Honey: Low pH for Health

The standard measure of the acidity or alkalinity of a solution is expressed as pH (potential of hydrogen). Aqueous solutions at 25°C (77°F) with a pH less than seven are considered acidic, whereas those with a pH greater than 7 are considered alkaline, or basic.

Honey is very acidic. Its pH is between 3 and 4, which is roughly the same pH as orange or grapefruit juice. Most types of bacteria thrive at pH levels between 7.2 and 7.4 and cannot survive at levels below pH 4.0, like those found in honey. But if the honey is diluted (for example, by the release of body fluids from a wound), it may become less acidic, allowing bacteria to grow again.

The low water activity of honey could be expected to dry out a wound, but this is not the case. The osmotic power of honey described above draws out fluid from the plasma or lymph in the tissues that underlie the wound. This activates the enzyme glucose oxidase, which enables the honey to produce hydrogen peroxide, an important factor in inhibiting bacterial growth and promoting immune activity.

Hydrogen Peroxide

Hydrogen peroxide is another reason why honey can heal. Hydrogen peroxide is created in the atmosphere when ultraviolet light strikes oxygen in the presence of moisture. When it comes into contact with water, this extra atom of oxygen splits off very easily. Water (H_2O) combines with the extra atom of oxygen and becomes hydrogen peroxide (H_2O_2).

Aside from being known as a powerful oxygenator and oxidizer, a special quality of hydrogen peroxide is its ability to readily decompose into water and oxygen. Hydrogen peroxide reacts easily with other substances and is able to kill bacteria, fungi, parasites, viruses, and even some types of tumor cells.

Hydrogen peroxide is involved in many of our body's natural processes. As an oxygenator, it is able to deliver small quantities of oxygen to the blood and other vital systems throughout the body. Hydrogen peroxide does not oxygenate the body merely by producing modest amounts of oxygen; it also has an extraordinary capacity to stimulate oxidative enzymes. Oxidative enzymes can change the chemical component of other substances (like viruses and bacteria) without being changed themselves. Rather than providing more oxygen to the cells, the presence of hydrogen peroxide enhances natural cellular oxidative processes, increasing the body's ability to use what oxygen is available.

Researchers have found that hydrogen peroxide must be present for our immune system to function properly. The cells in the body that fight infection (the class of white blood cells known as granulocytes) naturally produce hydrogen peroxide as a first line of defense against harmful parasites, bacteria, viruses, and fungi. Hydrogen peroxide is a hormonal regulator and is needed for the metabolism of protein, carbohydrates, fats, vitamins, and minerals. It is also a by-product of cell metabolism (that is actively broken down by peroxidase) and is necessary for the body's production of estrogen, progesterone, and thyroxin. If that wasn't enough, hydrogen peroxide is also involved in the regulation of blood sugar and the production of energy in body cells.[6]

Many of us have purchased 3 percent grade hydrogen peroxide in the pharmacy to disinfect wounds. However, some doctors have discouraged the use of hydrogen peroxide "out of the bottle" as a means for clearing more serious infections. Even at a 3 percent concentration, it can produce free radicals that can actually inhibit wound healing.

Hydrogen peroxide levels produced by diluted honey are approximately one thousand times lower that those in 3 percent hydrogen peroxide solutions. This low concentration may enable hydrogen peroxide to serve as an intracellular and intercellular "messenger" that stimulates wound healing without causing oxidative damage from free radicals.

H_2O_2 and Honey

I mentioned earlier that hydrogen peroxide is made naturally in honey by an enzyme called glucose oxidase, which is added to the plant nectar by the bee. Glucose oxidase is secreted from the hypopharyngeal gland of the bee into the nectar to help formulate honey from the nectar. It is believed that the hydrogen peroxide is used as a sterilizing agent during the honey's ripening process.

It's interesting to note that full-strength honey has a negligible level of hydrogen peroxide, because this substance is short-lived in the presence of the transition metal ions and ascorbic acid in honey, which cause the hygrogen peroxide to decompose to oxygen and water. Glucose oxidase has been found to be practically inactive in full-strength honey, giving rise to hydrogen peroxide only when the honey is diluted.

Dr. Katrina Brudzynski of the Department of Biological Sciences at Brock University in Ontario studied forty-two samples of Canadian honey to determine their antibacterial potential against strains of *Escherichia coli* and *Bacillus subtilis*. After tabulating the results, she concluded: "These data indicate that all Canadian honeys exhibited antibacterial activity, with higher selectivity against *E. coli* than *B. subtilis,* and that these antibacterial activities were correlated with hydrogen peroxide production in honeys. The hydrogen peroxide level in honey, therefore, is a strong predictor of the honey's antibacterial activity."[7]

When it comes to clearing infections, honey supplies low levels of hydrogen peroxide to wounds continuously over time as opposed to a large amount at the moment of treatment. In essence, it becomes a powerful yet effective "slow-release" antiseptic at a level that is antibacterial but does not damage tissue. In an article published in *Archives of Medical Research* on the activity of honey against medically significant bacteria carried out by members of the School of Biomedical Sciences at Charles Sturt University in Australia, the authors found: "The mild acidity and low-level hydrogen peroxide release assists both tissue repair and contributes to the antibacterial activity of honey. The antibacterial activity is a major factor in promoting wound healing where infection is present."[8]

Dilution with water has not been found to seriously inhibit hydrogen peroxide production in honey, an important factor to consider when treating exuding wounds. In a study carried out at the Honey Research Unit at the University of Waikato, eight honey samples from six different floral sources were tested. The maximum levels of accumulated hydrogen peroxide occurred in solutions diluted to concentrations of between 30 percent and 50 percent. The authors concluded: "Significant antibacterial activity can be maintained easily when using honey as a wound dressing, even on a heavily exuding wound."[9]

Pasteurization destroys the enzymes that produce hydrogen peroxide, so any honey used therapeutically should be raw and unpasteurized. The honey should be stored in a cool place and away from light. If it is necessary to liquefy the honey, it should be heated at a temperature no higher than 37°C (98.6°F).

Varying Antibacterial Potential

More than two thousand years ago, both Aristotle and Dioscorides recommended that honey collected in specific regions and seasons (and therefore presumably from different floral sources) be used for the treatment of particular ailments. Yet surprisingly, modern scientists didn't begin to compare the antibacterial potency of different honeys until about forty years ago.

They recognized that there are indeed differences in the antibacterial activity of different honeys, and a method was devised to determine the inhibine number of honeys as a measure of their antibacterial activity. The inhibine number is the degree of dilution to which a honey will retain its antibacterial activity, representing sequential dilutions of honey in steps of 5 percent from 5 percent to 25 percent. For example, one variety of honey may be able to kill a specific type of bacteria at a 15 percent dilution but not at 20 percent. Another honey can be diluted to 25 percent and still be effective at killing that same bacteria. The second honey would have a higher inhibine number.

Studies measuring the inhibine number of honeys have shown that antibacterial activity can vary considerably: up to a hundredfold. Some honeys are no more antibacterial than table sugar, while others can be strongly diluted and will be able to kill or inhibit the growth of bacteria.

Factors that influence antibacterial activity include not only the type of honey but also the region and specific area where it is collected: that is one reason, for example, why different samples of clover honey can vary in antibacterial activity. The honey's exposure to light during storage must also be considered. Plus, in some instances, honeys are simply misidentified, leading a person to believe that he or she is using one type of monofloral honey when in reality the person is using a honey derived from a different flower or from more than one flower source. Also, each honey type has a different inherent chemical stability that affects its antibacterial potential over time. The age of the honey at the time of use is also a factor: although honey never spoils, its effective therapeutic life usually extends for less than two years.

In a study of 345 samples of New Zealand honeys, 80 were found to have low antibacterial activity (36 percent of the samples had activity near or below the level of detection), with the rest having a distribution over nearly a twentyfold range of activity.[10] The major variations seen in overall antibacterial activity are due to different levels of hydrogen peroxide in different honeys. In some cases it was due to the level of nonperoxide factors, which I will discuss later on.

Hydrogen peroxide can be destroyed by several components of honey: it can be degraded by reaction with ascorbic acid and metal ions and by the action of catalase, an enzyme that comes from the pollen and nectar of certain plants, although more from the nectar. Also, differences have been found in the thermal stability of different honeys' glucose oxidase content and in the sensitivity of this hydrogen peroxide–producing enzyme to denaturation by light, because of a light-sensitizing component that comes from some floral sources. Scientists have also found that heating honey, which inactivates the glucose oxidase, causes loss of activity against some species of bacteria while it is retained against others.

Phytochemical Factors

While important, hydrogen peroxide activity does not account for all of honey's antibacterial activity. Honey also contains phytochemical factors, which are chemical compounds (such as a carotenoid or phytosterol) that occur naturally in plants. They are found in the nectar that the bees collect. Not only does each plant species supply specific phytochemicals, but the chemical activity can also vary from plant to plant.

In the past few years various researchers have identified an astonishing number of chemicals with antibacterial and antioxidant activity in honey, such as phenolics, peptides, organic acids, vitamins, and enzymes. Specifically, they include pinocembrin, terpenes, benzyl alcohol, 3,5-dimethoxy-4-hydroxybenzoic acid (syringic acid), methyl 3,5-dimethoxy-4-hydroxybenzoate (methyl syringate), 3,4,5-trimethoxy-benzoic acid, 2-hydroxy-3-phenylpropionic acid, 2-hydroxybenzoic acid, and 1,4-dihydroxybenzene.

Many of these chemical elements are beneficial to health. A study carried out by scientists at both the School of Applied Sciences at the University of Wales Institute in Cardiff and the Department of Biological Sciences at the University of Waikato found that both pasture honey and manuka honey stimulate the release of a variety of cytokines (immunoregulatory proteins that are secreted by cells, especially of the immune system). One of the most important of these cytokines is tumor necrosis factor, a protein that reduces tissue inflammation, induces the destruction of some tumor cells, and activates white blood cells, which is vital to healing.[11]

A laboratory study evaluating the antitumor activity of jungle honey, or JH (honey made by bees in the tropical forest the Nsukka area of Enugu state in Nigeria), was led by scientists of the Department of Biotechnology at the Kyoto Sangyo University in Japan. After infecting mice with lung cancer cells, they injected small amounts of JH solution daily into one group of mice, whereas the mice in the control group were left untreated. After seven days the incidence of cancerous tumors in the JH-injected mice was 20 percent, while that of the control group was 100 percent. In their report published in *Evidence Based Complementary and Alternative Medicine* in 2009, the researchers concluded that JH produces "potent antitumor activity." However, unlike manuka honey that contains tumor necrosis factor, they believe that phytochemical components in JH killed the tumors by stimulating the production of neutrophils (white blood cells that fight infection), which infiltrated the tumor tissue.[12]

In a study carried out by researchers at the Bloomberg School of Public Health at Johns Hopkins University in Baltimore, pinostrobin found in honey was able to induce mammalian phase-2 detoxification enzymes. These enzymes are part of a group of flavonoids (aromatic compounds found in certain plants that defend them from infection) believed to help protect humans against cancer and heart disease. After studying thirty-five types of honey, the researchers concluded that darker-colored varieties (such as buckwheat) were more potent inducers of pinostrobin than lighter varieties like acacia or sage. They commented: "Thus, the presence in honey of similarly acting phytochemicals, such as the flavonoids pinocembrin, pinostrobin, pinobanksin, and chrysin, makes this natural sweetener a logical source of dietary chemoprotective ability."[13]

The Antioxidant Capacity of Honey

Antioxidants are enzymes (such as catalase, superoxide dismutase, and glutathione peroxidase) that protect cells from free radicals by chemically changing them into harmless compounds like oxygen and water. Because excess free radical activity can seriously deplete our body's antioxidant reserves, nutritionists recommend that we augment those supplies with foods rich in antioxidants. Three common vitamins—beta-carotene (vitamin A), vitamin C, and vitamin E—are important dietary antioxidants, as are minerals like zinc and selenium.

These natural antioxidants can help inhibit or control excessive oxidation, in addition to protecting proteins, fats, and other substances in the body from oxidative damage. Antioxidants can also help stabilize cell membranes and have been found to influence chemical "messengers" both within and between body cells.

Many of the foods we eat—green and yellow vegetables, fruits, nuts, and seeds—contain antioxidant vitamins and minerals in abundance and are recommended as a major part of all healthy diets. Honey contains a variety of antioxidants as well, although in far smaller amounts than broccoli or oranges. Because honey is easily digested, some nutritionists have recommended it as an alternative to sugar and high-fructose corn syrup as a sweetener, because these products are devoid of antioxidants and other beneficial nutrients.

Honey Antioxidant Research

In a study undertaken by researchers at the Department of Food Sciences and Human Nutrition at the University of Illinois on the antioxidant components of honeys from eight American floral sources, most honeys were found to have similar but quantitatively different phenolic profiles. Buckwheat honey scored the highest of all honeys tested, followed by Hawaiian Christmas Berry, soy, tupelo, and clover honey. Fireweed and acacia honeys scored the lowest, with less than one-third the antioxidant activity of buckwheat and half of that of clover.

The researchers noted that the individual levels of a single phenolic or other antioxidant compound found in honey are too low to have a major individual antioxidant significance of their own. Yet the synergistic effects of the different compounds working together changed the picture considerably: ". . . the total antioxidant capacity of honey is likely the result of the combined activity and interactions of a wide range of compounds, including phenolics, peptides, organic acids, enzymes, Maillard reaction products, and possibly other minor components."[14]

A team of scientists at the National Research Center Dokki in Egypt studied the antioxidant activity of honey from four floral sources—two "light" varieties (acacia and coriander) and two "dark" honeys (sidr and palm)—to determine whether honey can inhibit oxidation of low-density lipoprotein (LDL), an early event in atherosclerosis. Atherosclerosis is the process in which deposits of fatty substances, cholesterol, cellular waste products, calcium, and other substances build up in the inner lining of an artery.

They found that while the darker varieties had higher antioxidant capacities, all varieties showed "highly effective" scavenging of the superoxide anion radical. When tested on LDL, the researchers found that "all honey samples (the darker and the lighter) and in all concentrations, were highly effective against LDL peroxidation."[15]

Their groundbreaking evidence suggests that it would be worthwhile to pursue in vivo studies on humans, which might prove that eating honey can help people reduce their LDL levels.

Which Honeys Have More Antibacterial Activity?

There are hundreds of varieties of honeys, and not enough research has been done to arrive at a final conclusion about the most "antibacterial" honey available today. One type of honey may be more effective against specific bacteria than others. For example, in a study undertaken at the University of Georgia, the researchers found that the growth of *S. sonnei,* a food-borne pathogen, was significantly more inhibited by Chinaso buckwheat honey than the other test varieties. By contrast, avocado honey scored higher in inhibiting the growth of *S. typhimurium,* another food-borne pathogen.[16]

Yet certain types of honey have been studied in large enough numbers for the following trends to be noted:

- Honeydew honey from the conifer forests of the mountainous regions of Germany and central Europe has been found to have particularly high antibacterial activity. In a study on the antibacterial activity of honey on *Helicobacter pylori,* the researchers found that Black Forest honey scored the highest among eight honeys in antibacterial activity.[17]
- Darker honeys (such as buckwheat, sidr, clover, manuka, ling heather, and borage) tend to have higher antibacterial activity than paler honeys like acacia, tawari, wild raspberry, and sage.

Two researchers from the Dr. ALM Post Graduate Institute of Basic Medical Sciences at the University of Madras in India tested manuka honey from Australia, heather honey from the United Kingdom, and two varieties of locally marketed Indian honey. They compared their antibacterial activity against fifty strains of *Pseudomonas aeruginosa* isolated from patients suffering from chronic suppurative otitis media, diabetic foot ulcers, and burn wound infections.

Using standard agar dilution methods, they found that the Minimum Inhibitory Concentrations (MICs) of different isolates of *Pseudomonas aeruginosa* were similar for manuka, heath, and local Indian honey (20 percent) while that of the locally produced raw Khadicraft brand honey scored substantially better at 11 percent.

Given the tendency to overlook the value of locally produced products, the authors concluded:

> Considering the enormous potential for the use of honey in a clinical setting, it is important that research continue not only using honeys that are commercially available but also with the locally available honeys. This study has shown that local products may have equal or sometimes better effectiveness than commercially available therapeutic honey.[18]

The Power of Manuka

One of the most exciting developments in the investigation of the phytochemical components of honey took place in 1988. This is when Dr. Peter C. Molan of the Department of Biological Sciences at the University of Waikato in New Zealand discovered that honey made from the flowers of New Zealand's manuka trees (*Leptospermum scoparium*) seems to be especially powerful at killing bacteria and doesn't depend on hydrogen peroxide activity to do so (figure 5.1). Although other honeys may well contain specific antibacterial properties, Dr. Molan believes that the antibacterial component found in *Leptospermum* plants is unique. That's why he decided to call it the Unique Manuka Factor (UMF) and developed a test to evaluate the UMF levels reflecting antibacterial strength as distinct from hydrogen peroxide activity.

Two discoveries have shed light on this mysterious "unique manuka factor." One, published in the November 2007 issue of the *Journal of Leucocyte Biology,* shows that there is a component of manuka honey (a protein known scientifically as 5.8-kDa) that stimulates immune cells

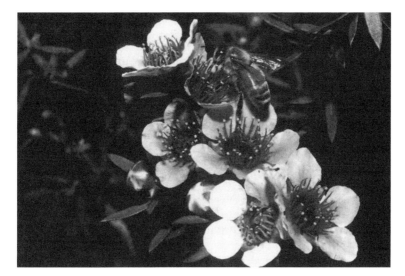

Figure 5.1. Honeybee visiting a manuka flower.
Photo courtesy of Peter C. Molan.

(including tumor necrosis factor described earlier) via the molecule TLR4, which is classified as a "toll-like receptor" that initiates cellular response and is believed to play a key role in the body's innate immune system.[19]

Methylglyoxal

Another discovery was reported in the journal *Carbohydrate Research* on January 12, 2008. A team of scientists in the Chemistry Department at the University of Waikato was able to isolate the fraction of New Zealand manuka honey that gives rise to its nonperoxide antibacterial activity. This fraction "proved to be methylglyoxal, a highly reactive precursor in the formation of advanced glycation endproducts (AGEs)."[20] Glycation (sometimes called nonenzymatic glycosylation) is the result of a sugar molecule, such as fructose or glucose, bonding to a protein or lipid molecule without the controlling action of an enzyme.

Writing in the January 21, 2008 issue of *Molecular Nutrition and Food Research,* Professor E. Mavric and colleagues of the Institute of Food Chemistry at the Technical University of Dresden reported the results of another study that "unambiguously demonstrates for the first time [actually, the second time] that methylglyoxal is directly responsible for the antibacterial activity of Manuka Honey." Researchers at the university analyzed forty samples of honey from various sources around the world, including six samples of New Zealand manuka honeys. They found methylglyoxal levels in manuka honeys were up to a thousandfold higher than nonmanuka products.[21]

However, the results of an earlier study published in the May 2006 issue of *Diabetes* caution that intracellular methylglyoxal "leads to an inhibition of insulin signaling." Thus "methylglyoxal may not only induce the debilitating complications of diabetes but may also contribute to the pathophysiology [the functional changes that accompany a particular syndrome or disease] of diabetes in general."[22]

Of course, the possibility of coming down with diabetes by ingesting honey that contains methylglyoxal depends on the individual patient, plus the amount of honey ingested over a given period of time. Nevertheless, this is one reason why physicians should differentiate among the different types of honey when recommending its internal use for patients with specific health problems.

The Properties of Manuka

UMF-rated Manuka honey has several outstanding healing properties. In laboratory tests UMF-rated Manuka honey inhibits the growth of *Heliobacter pylori,* a species of bacteria that is linked to stomach ulcers. It also kills *Citrobacter freundii, Escherichia coli, Proteus mirabilis,* and *Streptococcus faecalis.* The peroxide activity of other honeys (including ordinary manuka varieties) is not effective against these bacteria, which led Dr. Molan to conclude that manuka honey was superior to other honeys in treating infected wounds.[23]

Although both hydrogen peroxide and UMF-rated Manuka honey can totally inhibit the growth of *Staphylococcus aureus* during an eight-hour incubation period, manuka honey has been found to work twice as fast as the other honey varieties.[24]

UMF-rated Manuka honey is also significantly more effective than other honeys against *Streptococcus pyogenes,* which causes sore throats. It was also found to have a more potent antioxidant potential than other honey varieties and was able to completely quench added radicals within five minutes of spiking.[25]

The Testing Criteria

Manuka honey samples undergo two special tests developed by the Honey Research Unit at the University of Waikato before they can be classified as UMF-grade honey.

1. The first test is designed to reflect "Total Activity." A Total Activity rating shows all the antibacterial activity of the honey without distinguishing between enzyme activity (that produces hydrogen peroxide) or UMF activity. Any type of honey can have a Total Activity rating.

2. The second test is designed to reveal specific UMF activity in honey. After the Total Activity rating is established, catalase is added to the honey sample to destroy any enzyme activity. Then the UMF activity of the honey is measured, which can range from a rating of zero to twenty.

What Do the UMF Ratings Mean?

A rating of zero to four shows that the UMF factor is "not detectable," whereas a rating from five to ten shows that the honey can be used for "maintenance levels" only. Manuka honeys with UMF ratings of ten to fifteen are considered "useful" for most types of wound treatment, while those of fifteen and above are classified as "superior" by the Honey Research Unit. Manuka honey with a rating of ten or above is considered adequate for clinical use.

To prevent misuse of active manuka honey, a collective of producers known as the Active Manuka Honey Association (see the resources section) registered "UMF" as a trademark. Only licensed companies that meet specific criteria delineated by the Honey Research Unit and the AMHA can use both the name and trademark. At the time of this writing, the only lab approved and licensed to carry out UMF testing is

Gribbles Analytical Laboratories in Auckland, New Zealand. I mentioned how to identify genuine UMF-rated Manuka honey in chapter 2.

Medical Grade Manuka

In addition to the UMF rating, some manuka honey is classified as "medical grade" honey. Sold under brands like Apimed and Medihoney, it is made into a gel used primarily by health care providers for wound treatment. It is also the raw material for government-approved sterile dressings made up of active manuka honey and alginate fiber like the Apinate brand produced by Brightwake Ltd. in the United Kingdom. These products are officially classified as "medical devices" by the appropriate government agencies where the products are manufactured and/or sold.

Medical-grade honey goes through several important steps in collection, laboratory analysis, and processing. First, the raw honey is brought to the processor from accredited suppliers in new, unused, food-approved drums with tamperproof seals. A batch number is placed on each drum so that the finished product can be traced.

Once at the processing plant the honey is analyzed to determine its total activity, UMF rating, and levels of bacteria, yeast, and molds. If the honey is deemed not acceptable for medical grade, it is either classified as food grade or rejected completely.

The honey then undergoes minimal heat treatment to ensure that the active manuka content is unaffected, and then it goes through a fine-

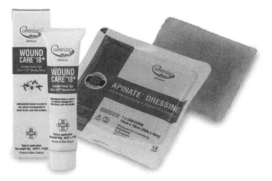

Figure 5.2. Comvita's honey-based medical products
Wound Care and Apinate Dressing

filtration process so that the standardized product contains less than 0.2 percent insoluble matter (by contrast, food-grade manuka honey can have 1 percent insoluble matter).

Sterilization of therapeutic honeys is achieved by gamma irradiation. Unlike the heat treatment used on supermarket honeys, which destroys the enzyme responsible for producing hydrogen peroxide,[26] gamma-irradiation does not hurt the antibacterial activity of either the hydrogen peroxide–type or the manuka "nonperoxide" honey in any way.[27] It ensures that the cfu/g (colony forming unit per gram) reading is less than 500 (food-grade manuka can have a maximum cfu/g of 100,000). Medical-grade honey is also tested for multipesticide residues (zero tolerance), moisture content, pH level, heavy metal content (zero tolerance), microbiological content, and other evaluations.[28]

The processed honey is then shipped to a licensed manufacturer that produces honey-based products like antiseptic creams and wound dressings. The manufacturer is certified with a CE* seal that reflects compliance with the highest standards of manufacture and testing for sales in Europe; or it will have certification by a reputable government agency in New Zealand, Australia, the United States, Canada, or other country.

Research continues to explore both the antioxidant and anti-inflammatory activities of honey. In the future, scientists will be able to better identify more of the specific components in honey that are responsible for these activities. In addition, they will be able to select honey that contains high levels of these activities for marketing and incorporate them into safe and effective medicines that can be used by doctors and patients around the world to treat a wide range of health problems.

---

*Officially, CE has no meaning as an abbreviation but may have originally stood for Communauté Européenne or Conformité Européenne, French for European Conformity.

6

HOW HONEY
TREATS WOUNDS

Honey has enormous potential to be a potent, nontoxic
treatment for wounds. . . . There is little doubt that honey
will be a valuable tool for all medical staff involved in the
management of wounds.

P. E. LUSBY, A. COOMBES AND J. M. WILKINSON;
SCHOOL OF BIOMEDICAL SCIENCES,
CHARLES STURT UNIVERSITY, AUSTRALIA

When Dr. Jennifer Eddy, a physician and professor of family medicine
at the University of Wisconsin Medical School at Eau Claire, first saw
the left foot of a seventy-nine-year-old man with type-2 diabetes, she was
shocked. The ulcer covering his forefoot was an unrecognizable black
mess. Most of the heel was a festering sore. Two of the man's toes had
been amputated, and he was unable to walk.

After five hospitalizations, four surgeries, and intense treatment with
antibiotics during the previous fourteen months—at a cost of $390,000—
the patient was considered a lost cause. Not only had he not responded
to antibiotic therapy, but the drugs were actually responsible for a variety
of medical complications, including acute kidney failure. His deep ulcers
were festering with MRSA, vancomycin-resistant *Enterococcus* (VRE), and

Pseudomonas, and it was only getting worse. Doctors wanted to amputate the patient's entire foot and told him he would most likely die unless they operated. The old man refused the operation but allowed the doctors to amputate a third toe before leaving the hospital and returning home.

With standard techniques exhausted, Eddy turned to a long-forgotten treatment used by physicians in ancient Egypt and Sumeria, prescribed by healers in India and China, and praised by Hippocrates and Galen: honey. Dr. Eddy carefully dressed the wounds in honey-soaked gauze and instructed members of the patient's family how to treat his wounds with honey at home. She described the man's course of treatment in her article appearing in the June 2005 issue of *The Journal of Family Practice.*

> Once daily, thick applications of ordinary honey purchased at a supermarket were smeared on gauze 4 x 4s and placed on the wounds, which were then wrapped. Oral antibiotics and saline dressings were discontinued, but otherwise treatment [for diabetes] was unchanged. Since the patient's family purchased and applied the honey, the cost of this therapy was merely that of the dressings. Dressing changes were painless and the serum glucose [blood glucose levels relating to diabetes] remained in excellent control.

The elderly man returned to Dr. Eddy every few weeks for evaluation. The results were astounding. Granulation (the growth of new tissue) began to appear in two weeks. Within six to twelve months, the ulcers completely healed. When Dr. Eddy wrote about her findings two years later, the ulcers had not reappeared. The patient was able to walk, and his overall quality of life had significantly improved.[1] Her experience with this elderly patient was not an isolated case. "I've used honey in a dozen cases since then," said Eddy. "I've yet to have one that didn't improve."[2]

Doctors Take Another Look

Physicians like Dr. Eddy have not only found that honey rapidly clears infections from wounds, but it also actually promotes healing. In the previous chapter I mentioned that laboratory studies have found that honey inhibits the growth of more than sixty types of bacteria, including those most commonly associated with wounds. It also works where bacteria-resistant antibiotics do not, such as killing the dreaded *Streptococcus pyogenes,* or "flesh-eating" bacteria. They've also found that honey rarely produces adverse side effects and is far more cost effective than traditional medicines used to treat both minor and serious wounds.

Why is honey such a miracle wound healer? Laboratory and clinical research offer the following reasons:

- Bacteria cannot live in the presence of honey. The osmotic pressure (pressure that sucks a solvent through a membrane of a cell into a denser solution) that honey naturally exerts removes water molecules from bacteria, making them shrivel up and die.
- Honey placed on a wound creates a physical barrier through which bacteria cannot pass.
- When honey is diluted with water, the glucose oxidase it contains becomes active and produces hydrogen peroxide, a powerful antibacterial agent.
- The sticky texture of honey prevents dried blood from adhering to the bandage. Dressings can be removed from the wound without hurting new skin cells.
- Adverse side effects of honey-based wound dressings are extremely rare.

What Kinds of Wounds Can Honey Treat?

Scientists at the Honey Research Unit at the University of Waikato in New Zealand have undertaken an ambitious program that now encompasses more than two-dozen different areas of investigation. These include developing a method to identify different honeys' floral sources by means of their chemical composition; assessing the antibacterial, antifungal, and immune-stimulating properties; investigating how the antimicrobial properties work against bacteria, fungi, and protozoa; conducting clinical trials on its effectiveness in treating wounds; and developing medical devices, treatment methods, and protocols for a variety of human and livestock diseases.

The author of dozens of articles appearing in peer-reviewed scientific and medical journals throughout the world, Dr. Peter Molan, the director of the Honey Research Unit, has assembled a database of literally hundreds of clinical findings on how honey can be used to treat the following wound conditions:

- abrasions
- amputations
- abscesses
- bed sores
- burst abdominal wounds following caesarian delivery
- cancrum oris (gangrenous ulcers of the mouth)
- cervical ulcers
- chilblains (inflamed swellings or sores caused by exposure to cold)
- cracked nipples
- cuts
- diabetic foot ulcers and other diabetic ulcers
- fistula
- foot ulcers in lepers
- infected wounds arising from trauma
- large septic wounds
- leg ulcers
- malignant ulcers
- sickle cell–related ulcers
- skin ulcers
- surgical wounds
- tropical ulcers
- wounds to the abdominal wall and perineum
- varicose ulcers[3]

Writing in the journal *Annals of Medicine,* Philip C. Bowler observed, "In order to maximize the opportunity for wound healing it is necessary to create conditions in the local environment that are favorable to the host repair mechanisms and unfavorable to micro-organisms."[4]

Honey works in a variety of significant ways to help the body fight off wound infection and make it difficult for harmful microorganisms to survive. It also possesses unique properties that enable the patient to feel more comfortable on both physical and psychological levels.

Antibacterial Activity

In the previous chapter I discussed how honey kills viruses, fungi, and bacteria. This is accomplished by the production of low yet constant levels of hydrogen peroxide that both inhibit bacteria and stimulate the human immune system.

I also mentioned how honey kills pathogens by the myriad phytochemicals it contains. These chemicals are found in the nectar collected by the bees and include various types of phenolics, peptides, organic acids, vitamins, and enzymes. Other plant-derived factors have yet to be identified. Honey from floral sources like *Leptospermum scoparium* (manuka) and *Leptospermum polygalifolium* (an Australian plant whose honey is marketed commercially as Medihoney) have been found to possess additional antioxidant, antibacterial, or other healing factors. Medihoney bears the CE seal (compliance certification) for medical products, and its quality is regularly tested.

Other types of honeys may well contain unidentified phytochemical factors as well. Because forward-looking scientists and drug companies in New Zealand and Australia have recognized both the healing and the commercial potential of these two *Leptospermum*-based honeys, these honeys have been subjected to extensive research. Other individual honeys have not yet been studied to the same extent.

Honey and Emergency First Aid

Because its strong antibacterial ability quickly renders even heavily infected wounds sterile without the use of antibiotics, honey is a perfect first-aid dressing.

It is especially useful for patients living in remote areas that are far from a physician or hospital. Because infection can easily set in when wounds are left untreated, emergency application of honey to a wound or burn will keep the wound sterile until it can receive proper medical attention.

Enhanced Immune System Activity

In addition to its direct action on bacteria and other pathogens, honey also promotes healing through its effect on the immune system.

Honey at concentrations as low as 1 percent has been found to stimulate the proliferation of peripheral blood B-lymphocytes and T-lymphocytes (two kinds of white blood cells that helps defend the body from disease) in cell culture and active phagocytes (cells that ingest bacteria) from blood. These cells activate the body's natural immune system to fight infection.

And at even a 1 percent concentration, honey can stimulate monocytes (another type of white blood cell) in cell culture and release cytokines (proteins that regulate both the intensity and duration of immune response) including tumor necrosis factor-1, interleukin-1, and interleukin-6.[5]

Deodorization

One of the most psychologically debilitating aspects of an infected wound is the strong odor. This is caused by malodorous substances produced by bacteria, including ammonia, sulfur compounds, and certain types of amino acids. On one level, honey kills the anaerobic bacteria (bacteria that thrive in a low-oxygen environment) found in chronic wounds, including *Bacteroides* spp., *Peptostreptococcus* spp., and *Prevotella* spp. In addition, honey contains copious amounts of glucose, a substrate (a substance acted upon and changed by an enzyme) metabolized by bacteria in preference to amino acids. This is why honey can deodorize wounds so rapidly and effectively.[6] In some cases where wounds grow exuberantly like a fungus, honey was found to be the only way to control the offensive odor.[7]

Many patients suffering from chronic wounds are not only psychologically debilitated by what they can smell but also are convinced that everyone around them can smell the unpleasant odor. This can severely impact their overall quality of life, including limiting their professional and social activities.

There have been numerous reported cases of how honey applications either reduce or eliminate wound odor. Writing in the text *Honey: A Modern Wound Management Product,* Val Robson, Lee Martin, and Rose Cooper relate the case history of a young woman with a serious breast infection that did not respond to antibiotics. The patient found both the lack of healing and accompanying odor very distressing to the point that she refused to look at the wound and would only allow her mother to change the dressings.

After two weeks of treatment with sterile dressings made with

Medihoney, the dead tissue from the wound cleared up and was replaced by healthy tissue. The patient rejoiced that the malodor was also completely resolved, adding that the odor control resulting from the use of honey was of "paramount importance" to her. After eleven weeks, the woman reported that the wound was completely healed.[8]

Wound Debridement

Like other moist wound dressings, honey facilitates the debridement—or the removal of dead tissue and foreign matter—from a wound. It accomplishes this feat through the process of autolysis, or the digestion of cells by different types of enzymes.

I mentioned earlier that honey produces strong osmotic activity by drawing out lymph fluid from wound tissues. This helps to kill bacteria, because bacteria need liquid to grow. At the same time, honey serves as a protective barrier to the crossinfection of wounds.

This osmotic action also provides a constantly replenished supply of proteases (also known as proteolytic enzymes) that also aids in wound debridement. Dr. Molan found that honey also has the ability to "wash" the surface of the wound bed from below, which aids in the removal of dirt and grit. It also helps separate dead tissue from the wound and allows granulation—the formation of small connective tissue projections as part of the healing process—to occur.

In addition, osmosis prevents the new tissue from becoming too soft due to an accumulation of moisture. According to Dr. Molan: "The osmotic action of honey also removes any risk of skin surrounding a wound becoming macerated [softened] by the moisture accumulating under a dressing. Even when diluted, honey will induce a withdrawal of moisture rather than a hydration of skin."[9]

When honey is placed on a wound, osmosis creates a layer of fluid beneath the bandage made up of the honey diluted in plasma or lymph. This makes it impossible for the bandage to adhere to the wound. When the dressing is removed, new-growth tissue isn't torn away.

Anti-inflammatory Action

Although inflammation is the normal response to injury, prolonged or excessive inflammation can inhibit the healing process. In addition to reducing patient discomfort, reducing inflammation helps reduce the size of the blood vessels within the wound and reduces edema and exudate, the fluid that exudes from an infected wound. Pressure in tissues caused by edema can restrict the flow of blood through the capillaries, starving the tissues of oxygen and nutrients that are needed to heal.

Both laboratory and clinical studies have proved honey's ability to reduce wound inflammation, especially in skin ulcers and both deep and surface burns. The antioxidant content of honey, which helps get rid of free radical activity, is seen as a factor in this healing effect. Commenting on the clinical evidence that shows honey's effectiveness in treating burn wounds, Dr. Molan wrote, "Honey's significant antioxidant content mops up free radicals, which might explain why, in one study, honey dressings prevented partial-thickness burns from converting to full-thickness burns."[10]

Reduced Scarring

Long-term infection can lead to the development of scars. Dr. Molan reports that the anti-inflammatory action of honey "provides the most likely explanation for the reduction of hypertrophic scarring [scarring characterized by an increase of hard, raised tissue] observed in wounds that were dressed with honey."[11]

New Tissue Growth

Honey has been proved clinically to stimulate tissue growth in a variety of wounds, including skin ulcers and burns. Honey also can stimulate collagen synthesis, which involves the formation of connective tissue, cartilage, and bone. Honey has also been found to stimulate angiogenesis—the development of new blood vessels—in wounds. This increases oxygen supply to the wound and supplies essential nutrients to the fibroblasts involved in collagen formation.

I mentioned earlier that honey promotes the formation of clean, healthy granulation tissue. This is accomplished in part by supplying glucose to the epithelial cells. These skin-producing cells must build up an internal store of carbohydrate, which provides the energy the cells need to migrate across the surface of a wound.[12] This migration eventually leads to the formation of new skin, known clinically as re-epithelialization. This promotion of skin growth is why honey is often used to treat patients suffering from burns and those receiving skin grafts.

In 1998 the medical journal *Burns* published the results of a randomized controlled clinical trial that compared the effectiveness of silver sulfadiazine (SSD)—a topical antimicrobial agent used commonly in the treatment of burns—and honey (the type of honey was not identified). Eighty-four percent of the patients treated with honey showed satisfactory epithelialization after seven days, with 100 percent after twenty-one days. By contrast, only 72 percent of those treated with SSD showed satisfactory healing by the seventh day, and only 84 percent experienced complete epithelialization by the twenty-first day.[13]

Honey: The Downsides

Although honey has numerous advantages over other treatments in wound healing, it's important to mention that it has several disadvantages as well.

1. Honey can become more fluid at higher temperatures. It may liquefy at wound temperature, thus making it less effective.
2. The risk of liquefaction can cause leakage and create a terrible mess.
3. Preparation of homemade honey dressings is not easy.
4. A small number of patients (approximately 5 percent) have experienced a temporary stinging sensation in the wound, which is a major cause of discomfort.

The availability of commercially produced sterile dressings impregnated with honey (such as Medihoney prepared gels and dressings, Activon

Tulle, and Comvita's Apinate dressing) enable health care practitioners to avoid many of these problems. Some of these new dressings contain a hard gel that swells to a softer gel as it absorbs liquid from the wound. This enables the honey to keep in contact with the wound itself, while preventing the moisture from leaving the bandaged area. I provide Dr. Molan's guidelines for using homemade honey dressings in the following chapter, which should help minimize some of these problems.

The clinical evidence for the use of honey as a safe, effective, and inexpensive wound treatment is accumulating steadily. In addition to laboratory research on the therapeutic aspects of honey, many hospitals and universities have undertaken clinical research, documenting the treatment of actual wound patients. Although an entire book could be devoted to the aspect of honey in wound healing alone, the following chapter features some of the most important studies.

7

THE CLINICAL
EVIDENCE

*Honey is the most ancient wound dressing known, but as
a bioactive dressing material it is also the most modern
type of wound dressing.*

PETER C. MOLAN,
PROFESSOR OF BIOLOGICAL SCIENCES
AND DIRECTOR OF THE HONEY RESEARCH UNIT,
UNIVERSITY OF WAIKATO, NEW ZEALAND

Franklin Lloyd, a retired attorney from Queens, New York, first noticed
that his right leg was swollen in December 2007. Originally diagnosed
with bacterial cellulitis, doctors eventually discovered a serious fungal
infection caused by *Cryptococcus* yeast. Traditional treatment (veracono-
zol) was not able to heal the infection, so another medication was used.
Although successful, the treatment left Mr. Lloyd with a "huge ulcerated
wound" encompassing most of the calf of his right leg, making it impossible for him to walk. Believing that there was no way the wound could
heal, doctors at the North Shore University Hospital in Manhasset, New
York, considered amputating Lloyd's leg just below the knee.

Yet thanks to a suggestion by clinical nurse specialist Mary Brennan,
his physician decided to use Medihoney on the wound, and within one

month, there was "significant improvement." After less than a year of honey treatment and physical therapy, Lloyd was eventually able to regain use of his leg.[1] His hospital news conference in January 2009 was carried by newspapers and television throughout the New York area, calling attention to the amazing effectiveness of this simple four-thousand-year-old remedy.

Since the 1980s, physicians, biochemists, and other scientists have been studying the values of honey for wound healing extensively in hospitals, universities, and other research centers primarily in Europe, India, and Asia. Although the medical literature documents more than a hundred cases, I present only a representative selection of them here.

Chronic Wounds Resistant to Healing

One of the earliest clinical trials in the medicinal use of honey was undertaken by researchers at the University Teaching Hospital in Calabar, Nigeria, and reported in the *British Journal of Surgery* in 1988. A total of fifty-nine patients suffering from recalcitrant wounds and ulcers took part in the trial, including forty-seven who had been treated unsuccessfully with traditional antibiotics for what clinicians called a "sufficiently long time." The wounds were varied and included Fournier's gangrene, cancrum oris, diabetic ulcers, traumatic ulcers, sickle-cell ulcers, and tropical ulcers. All were treated with honey. One patient, suffering from a Buruli ulcer (a severe and stubborn tropical skin infection caused by *Mycobacterium ulcerans*), did not respond to therapy, while the fifty-eight others "showed remarkable improvement following topical application of honey," with infected wounds becoming sterile within one week.[2]

A more recent randomized controlled trial (a prospective experiment in which investigators randomly assign an eligible sample of patients to one or more treatment groups and a control group and then follow the patients' outcomes) was carried out by leg-ulcer specialists at the Aintree University Hospitals in Liverpool, England. A sample of 105 patients was treated with either standardized antibacterial honey (Medihoney) or conventional wound dressings between September 2004 and May 2007.

The results were impressive: the median healing time in the group treated with honey was 100 days compared to 140 days for the group receiving traditional therapy. The physicians also found that the healing rate at twelve weeks was equal to 46.2 percent in the honey group and 34.0 percent in the conventional group. While the clinicians felt that further research is needed, they wrote: "These results support the proposition that there are clinical benefits from using honey in wound care."[3]

Pressure Ulcers

A pressure ulcer is an area of skin that breaks down when you stay in one position for too long without shifting your weight. This often happens if you use a wheelchair or are bedridden. A pressure ulcer can appear even after a short period of time, such as after surgery or an injury. The constant pressure against the skin reduces the blood supply to that area, and the affected tissue dies. Millions of people suffer from pressure ulcers each year.

Two research professors at the Ege University School of Nursing in Izmir, Turkey, evaluated the effectiveness of a honey dressing for healing pressure ulcers. They selected sixty-eight patients for the study: fifteen patients with twenty-five pressure ulcers were treated with honey dressings made from raw, natural organic, and unpasteurized honey that was sterilized by exposure to gamma irradiation. Eleven patients with twenty-five pressure ulcers were treated with ethoxy-diaminoacridine plus nitrofurazone dressings, a standard treatment for pressure ulcers. Both groups were statistically similar regarding baseline and wound characteristics. Wound healing was assessed weekly using the PUSH tool: a standardized method designed to evaluate pressure ulcers.

After five weeks of treatment, patients who were treated with honey had significantly better PUSH-tool scores than subjects treated with the ethoxy-diaminoacridine plus nitrofurazone dressings. The researchers concluded: "By week 5, PUSH tool scores showed that healing among subjects using a honey dressing was approximately 4 times the rate of healing in the comparison group. The use of a honey dressing is effective and practical."[4]

Postsurgical Wounds

The usefulness of honey dressings as an alternative method of managing abdominal surgical wounds was assessed in a two-year clinical trial at Ramathibodi Hospital, which is part of Mahidol University in Bangkok, Thailand. Fifteen patients whose wounds disrupted after undergoing caesarian section were treated with honey application and wound dressing by micropore tape instead of the conventional method of subsequent resuturing. A control group of nineteen patients had its wounds cleaned with hydrogen peroxide and Dakin solution and packed with saline-soaked gauze prior to resuturing under general anesthesia.

The results were impressive. Researchers noted that among the patients treated with honey dressings, slough (dead tissue separating living tissue from an ulcer) and necrotic (dead) tissue were replaced by granulation (new tissue) and advancing epithelialization (scabbing) within two days. Foul-smelling wounds were made odorless within one week. Excellent results were achieved in all the cases treated with honey, thus avoiding the need to resuture, a procedure requiring general anesthesia.

Among members of the group treated with honey, eleven of the cases were completely healed within seven days, and all were healed within two weeks. The period of hospitalization was two to seven days (mean 4.5 days), compared with nine to eighteen days (mean 11.5 days) for members of the control group. Two patients in the control group experienced reinfection, and one patient developed jaundice from the anaesthetic. The researchers concluded, "We achieved excellent results in all the cases with complete healing within 2 weeks. Honey application is inexpensive, effective and avoids the need to resuture, which also requires general anesthesia."[5]

Another study on postoperative wound infection was carried out by physicians at the General Private Hospital in Sana'a, Yemen, and reported in the *European Journal of Medical Research*. Fifty patients suffering from postoperative wound infections following caesarian sections or total abdominal hysterectomies with bacterial infections were allocated in two groups. Twenty-six patients (group A) were treated with twelve hourly applications of raw, unfiltered honey a day, and twenty-four patients (group B) were given local antiseptics, including 70 percent ethanol and povidone-iodine. Members of both groups received systemic antibiotics according to the culture and sensitivity of their wound.

Results showed that the patients treated with honey (group A) experienced a complete healing of bacterial infections in half the time as members of the control group (group B). The average size of their postoperative scars was less than half the size of those of the controls, and the average length of hospitalization was 75 percent shorter as well. After using honey twenty-two of the twenty-six patients (84.4 percent) in group A showed complete wound healing without wound disruption or need for resuturing, and only four patients showed mild dehiscence (re-opening of the surgical wound). In group B, twelve of twenty-four patients (50 percent) showed complete wound healing, and the other twelve patients showed wound dehiscence. Six of them needed resuturing under general anesthesia.

The researchers concluded that topical application of crude undiluted honey could result in faster eradication of bacterial infections, reduction of the period of antibiotic use and hospital stay, acceleration of wound healing, prevention of wound dehiscence (and need for resuturing), and minimization of scar formation.[6]

A review article in the October 2007 issue of the *International Journal of Clinical Practice* examined both the nutritional value and the broad range of clinical applications of honey. The three physicians who wrote the article were so impressed with honey's ability to fight postsurgical infection that they concluded: "The use of honey in the surgical wards is highly recommended and patients about to undergo surgery should ask their surgeons if they could apply honey to the wounds postoperation."[7]

Studies among Cancer Patients

Medical experts from the University of Bonn in Germany have documented their largely positive experience with treating wounds with honey. Even chronic wounds infected with multiresistant bacteria often healed within a few weeks. One of the most promising aspects of honey treatment is that it excels against bacteria that are often resistant to traditional antibiotics. According to Dr. Arne Simon, who works at the cancer ward at the university's Children's Clinic, "In hospitals today we are faced with germs [that] are resistant to almost all the current antibiotics. As a result, the medical use of honey is becoming attractive again for the treatment of wounds."

As far as wound treatment is concerned, his young patients form part of a high-risk group: chemotherapy (also known as cytostatics) to treat cancer not only slows down the reproduction of malignant cells but also impairs the healing process of wounds. "Normally a skin injury heals in a week: with our children it often takes a month or more," Dr. Simon explains. Moreover, children with leukemia have a weakened immune system. If a germ enters their bloodstream via a wound, the result may be a fatal case of blood poisoning.[8]

German pediatricians are pioneers for the use of Medihoney in treating wounds. "The success is astonishing: 'Dead tissue is rejected faster, and the wounds heal more rapidly,' Dr. Kai Sofka, a wound specialist at the University Children's Clinic, emphasizes. 'What is more, changing dressings is less painful, since the poultices are easier to remove without damaging the newly formed layers of skin. Even wounds [that] consistently refused to heal for years can, in our experience, be brought under control with medihoney. And this frequently happens within a few weeks.'"[9] At the present time, at least two-dozen hospitals in Germany are routinely using honey to treat wounds.

A study at Aintree Hospital in Liverpool, England, evaluated *Leptospermum* honey's ability to manage wounds in which healing was impaired by radiotherapy. Four patients from sixty-three to ninety-three years of age were evaluated: all had undergone radiotherapy that left them with damaged skin that did not respond to conventional treatment. Compromised areas included the neck, cheek, groin/perineum, and chest. The researchers reported that

> in patients 1 and 2, after topical application of honey via hydrofiber rope and nonadhesive foam, respectively, improvements in the size and condition of the wound/periwound area and a reduction in pain were noted before death [patient 1] or loss to follow-up [patient 2]. After including honey in the treatment regimen of patients 3 and 4, complete healing was noted in 2.5 weeks (with honey and paraffin) and 6 weeks (with honey-soaked hydrofiber rope), respectively.

They concluded: "Honey as an adjunct to conventional wound/
skin care post radiation therapy shows promise for less painful healing in these chronic wounds."[10]

A study by three physicians at the division of Radiotherapy and
Oncology at the School of Medical Sciences, Universiti Sains Malaysia
evaluated the effect of natural honey on radiation-induced mucositis,
which is inflammation of the mucous membranes due to radiation.

Forty patients diagnosed with head and neck cancer requiring radiation were divided into two groups. The controls received radiation alone,
while the other group received radiation and topical applications of natural raw honey. Patients were evaluated every week for eleven months.

The researchers found that there was a significant reduction in symp-
tomatic mucositis among honey-treated patients: only 20 percent suffered
from this problem as opposed to 75 percent of the controls. The doctors
concluded: "Topical application of natural honey is a simple and cost-
effective treatment in radiation mucositis, which warrants further multi-
center randomized trials to validate our finding."[11]

A systematic review of forty-three studies of the use of honey in wound
healing and its potential value within oncology care was undertaken
by four researchers at several hospitals and universities in Manchester,
England. Their findings, published in the *Journal of Clinical Nursing* in
October 2008, highlighted the need for randomized controlled trials. Yet
the authors concluded: "Honey was found to be a suitable alternative for
wound healing, burns and various skin conditions and to potentially have
a role within cancer care."[12]

Meningococcal Septicemia

One of the most dramatic case studies—which was picked up by the
media—was first reported in the April 2000 issue of the British journal *Nursing Times* by Cheryl Dunford, lecturer in tissue viability at the
School of Nursing and Midwifery, Southampton University. It concerned
a fifteen-year-old boy named "Jem" who suffered from a severe case of
meningococcal septicemia, which led to high levels of blood toxicity.

This not only led to adult respiratory distress syndrome and renal failure but also the amputation of both hands and feet due to tissue necrosis. Multiple skin grafts were harvested and applied to what was left of his limbs; however, the grafts on his legs did not heal even after six months and caused Jem unbearable pain.

Despite intensive medical therapy, infection was rampant (primarily with *Pseudomonas* spp., *Staphylococcus aureus,* and *Enterococcus* spp.), and traditional treatments with antibiotics and different types of dressings proved ineffective. Because of the severe pain, dressing changes had to be done every three days under general anesthesia.

Clinicians finally introduced absorbent dressing pads impregnated with 25 to 35g of UMF-13 Manuka honey to the right leg (the left leg was treated with traditional antibiotics as a control). Within a few days the right leg showed signs of epithelialization with a corresponding reduction in bacteria, especially the *Pseudomonas* and *Enterococcus.* Honey was then used on all skin lesions on both legs, with continued epithelialization; new skin grafts were applied and proved successful after many failed attempts. Jem's pain lessened considerably, and dressing changes were done without general anesthesia. Dr. Dunford reported:

> Within ten weeks all lesions, including the pressure ulcer, were completely healed and Jem was able to be discharged and to begin his very successful rehabilitation program. Not only did the lesions finally heal within a relatively short period of time, but also the resultant scar tissue was of good quality with no evidence of hyper-tropic scarring.[13]

Honey and Milk against *Staphylococcus aureus* Infection

Like honey, both cow and human milk were found to possess antimicrobial properties. The mixture of warm milk and honey has been a popular remedy for insomnia and gastrointestinal problems for centuries, and mothers throughout the Middle East often give it to their children on a daily basis.

Dr. A. A. Al-Jabri and colleagues at the College of Medicine and Health Sciences at Sultan Qaboos University in Oman tested the antibacterial properties of bovine milk alone and in combination with various samples of Omani honey on *Staphylococcus aureus*. Measuring the percentage growth inhibition of *S. aureus* by honey alone, milk alone, and in combination at various time points in a twenty-four-hour period, they found that a combination of milk and honey was more effective in inhibiting bacterial growth than either honey alone or milk alone (milk alone wasn't effective at all). Writing in the *British Journal of Biomedical Science,* they concluded: "Although the exact mechanisms by which honey in combination with milk acts against *S. aureus* remains unclear, it is possible that honey releases some of the biogenic peptides in milk that have an antimicrobial effect. Clearly, this enhanced effect is important and is an area that requires more research."[14]

Herpes

A study undertaken by Dr. Noori S. Al-Waili, director of the Dubai Specialized Medical Center and Medical Research Laboratories in the United Arab Emirates compared the effect of the topical application of honey to acyclovir cream on recurrent attacks of labial and genital herpes lesions. It was the first in vivo study on the antiviral qualities of honey and garnered much interest among physicians in developing countries, where herpes medicines like acyclovir cream are very expensive and beyond the reach of most patients.

He started with a group of sixteen adult patients that had a history of recurrent attacks of herpes lesions. Eight patients suffering from labial herpes and eight patients diagnosed with genital herpes were treated with a topical application of honey for one attack and with acyclovir cream for another attack.

For patients with labial herpes, the mean duration of attacks and pain, occurrence of crusting, and mean healing time with honey treatment were 35 percent, 39 percent, 28 percent, and 43 percent better, respectively, than with acyclovir treatment. For those with genital herpes, the mean duration of attacks and pain, occurrence of crusting, and mean healing time with honey treatment were 53 percent, 50 percent, 49 percent, and 59 percent shorter, respectively, than with acyclovir.

Dr. Al-Waili also found that two cases of labial herpes and one case of genital herpes remitted completely with the use of honey. The lesions crusted in three patients with labial herpes and in four patients with genital herpes. With acyclovir treatment, none of the attacks remitted and all the lesions, labial and genital, developed crust.

No side effects were observed with repeated applications of honey, whereas three patients developed local itching with acyclovir. Dr. Al-Waili concluded that "topical honey application is safe and effective in the management of the signs and symptoms of recurrent lesions from labial and genital herpes."[15]

Dr. Al-Waili's study led Dr. Arne Simon and colleagues at the Children's Hospital Medical Centre at the University of Bonn to routinely treat children and adults with recurrent herpetic lip lesions with medical honey. Dr. Simon also reports: "We use topical medical honey in addition to systemic acyclovir in immunocompromised patients with [herpes] zoster to prevent secondary bacterial skin infection and to accelerate healing of the herpetic lesions."[16]

Research among Gold Miners

Doctors from the Department of Family Medicine at the University of Limpopo (Medunsa Campus) carried out a recent double-blind study comparing honey and the popular branded wound dressing IntraSite Gel among gold mine workers in South Africa. Outcome criteria included healing times of shallow wounds and abrasions, side effects, patient satisfaction with treatment, and the amount of honey and IntraSite Gel used.

The researchers found that the mean healing times of shallow wounds treated with honey or with IntraSite Gel did not differ significantly. When adjusted for wound size, the 2.8-day difference in favor of honey was considered clinically insignificant. In the case of abrasions, there was no significant difference either. When adjusted for wound size, the difference of 0.22 days in favor of IntraSite Gel was also considered statistically insignificant.

Side effects varied. Among the patients treated with honey, 27 percent experienced itching, 10 percent experienced pain, and 2 percent felt a burning sensation for a short time after application. Among those treated with IntraSite Gel, 31 percent experienced itching, but none felt pain or burning. All patients in both treatment groups were either "satisfied" or "extremely satisfied" with treatment.

The main difference involved the average cost per patient treatment: one treatment with honey cost .49 South African Rand (ZAR) (approximately $.07 USD), whereas one treatment with IntraSite Gel cost 12.03 ZAR (approximately $1.66 USD). The researchers concluded: "There was no evidence of a real difference between honey and IntraSite Gel as healing agents. Honey is a safe, satisfying and effective healing agent. Natural honey is extremely cost effective."[17]

Studies with Patented Honey Dressings

A 2003 study by Dr. Jackie Stephen-Haynes and her colleagues at the Worcestershire Primary Care Trusts and University College in Worcester, England, involved evaluating treatment of twenty patients with a variety of wounds. Clinicians treated the wounds with Activon Tulle, a sterile, nonadherent dressing impregnated with medical-grade New Zealand manuka honey, described later in this chapter. Dr. Stephen-Haynes observed "medical grade honey does appear to be a valuable addition to the wound management formulary."[18]

Proffessor Cheryl Dunford, who evaluated the effects of honey dressings on patients with leg ulcers, focusing particularly on pain, odor, and patient satisfaction, undertook a more recent British study. She concluded that the honey dressings were not only clinically effective but also produced a high level of patient satisfaction. However, she recommended further clinical trials to evaluate how honey compares to traditional wound dressings.[19]

As a nurse at the Woodfield Retirement Village near Sydney, Australia, Elizabeth van der Weyden has treated many elderly patients suffering from a wide range of health problems. One of her patients was a man suffering from venous leg ulcers that did not respond to traditional antibiotics. She decided to use a honey-impregnated alginate dressing (a pharmaceutical dressing derived from green algae that cleanses wounds and keeps them moist) as an alternative treatment, which continued for several weeks. In an article appearing in the *British Journal of Community Nursing* she concluded, "The honey seemed to act as an effective antibacterial, anti-inflammatory and deodorizing dressing, with total healing of the ulcer achieved. This result, together with past successes with the use of honey alginate on ulcerated wounds, has led to this product becoming main-stream in the treatment of chronic wounds within our care facility."[20]

While promising, these reports show that more randomized clinical trials are needed to compare commercially prepared honey dressings with traditional antibiotics in treating wounds.

After Nail Bed Surgery

A joint study carried out by researchers at the University of Huddersfield and the University of Edinburgh compared healing times between manuka-impregnated honey dressings and paraffin tulle gras (a soft dress-ing consisting of open-woven silk or other material impregnated with a waterproof soft paraffin wax) following toenail surgery. One hundred patients took part in the double-blind study to evaluate the length of time it took for complete reepithelialization of the nail bed to occur. Each patient was seen twice a week for examination and dressing change.

The results were statistically similar: mean healing times for the patients treated with honey was 40.39 days, whereas those treated with paraffin tulle gras was 38.98 days. Patients with partial nail removal did better with paraffin tulle, while those with complete toenail removal had better results with honey. Although the researchers concluded that patients would benefit more from the paraffin tulle dressings, they wrote: "The marginal benefit of the honey dressing on these healing times war-rants further investigation."[21]

MRSA-infected Wounds

Although laboratory tests have documented the ability of honey to kill a wide variety of superbugs, few clinical studies have been done. And none have been the double-blind studies considered the "gold standard" of medical research.

One of the first articles to document the effectiveness of honey on MRSA-colonized leg ulcers was written by Dr. Subramanian Natarajan and colleagues at the University of Wales College of Medicine and published in the *Journal of Dermatological Treatment* in 2001. They reported the case of an immunosuppressed patient who developed a hydroxyurea-induced leg ulcer with a subclinical MRSA infection. They treated this patient with a topical application of manuka honey, while continuing treatment with hydroxyurea and cyclosporin. The MRSA was completely eradicated from the ulcer, and rapid healing was successfully achieved.[22]

An article appearing in the September 2007 issue of the *Journal of Wound Care* examined the effects of honey-impregnated dressings on MRSA-infected wounds. The results were compiled by clinicians at the Children's Hospital Medical Center of the University of Bonn.

They found that complete healing was achieved in seven consecutive patients whose wounds were either infected or colonized with MRSA. Antiseptics and antibiotics had previously failed to eradicate the clinical signs of infection.

In this study, all patients were treated with Medihoney antibacterial medical honey. In accordance with the internal wound-care standard for the use of antibacterial medical honey at the hospital, the dressings were changed daily by a professional wound-care nurse or a trained relative when patients were being cared for at home. The results greatly impressed the researchers, because MRSA infections are notoriously difficult to treat. They developed a database (known as the Woundpecker Database) for the standardized collection of data on the clinical use of Medihoney products in wound care, with a view to fostering the collection of clinical evidence and to perform prospective comparative studies in the future. The researchers concluded: "These results should encourage others to use CE certified antibacterial honey dressings in wounds infected or colonized with MRSA. Nonetheless, prospective randomized studies are urgently needed to confirm the real benefit of this unconventional treatment approach."[23]

Which Honey Is Best for Wound Healing?

In chapter 5 I mentioned that honey produced from different flower sources will have varying degrees of antibacterial activity. In ancient Greece, the noted physician Dioscorides recommended a pale yellow honey from Attica as best for wound healing, whereas Aristotle (384–322 BCE) referred to pale honey as being "good as a salve for sore eyes and wounds."

Today, honey from Sardinia's strawberry tree is highly regarded for its therapeutic properties, while honey from Yemen's Jirdin Valley is especially revered by folk healers in neighboring Dubai. Traditional Russian healers have found that buckwheat, sweet clover, white, and chestnut honeys produce strong antibacterial effects and recommend them for wound healing. Raw, unfiltered tupelo honey is preferred by folk healers in Florida.

I mentioned earlier that in New Zealand wound-care specialists have long preferred manuka honey, the subject of intense scientific scrutiny because of its unusual healing powers. Coming from the native manuka bush (*Leptospermum scoparium*) that grows wild on undeveloped, unspoiled, and regenerating land, its leaves and flowers possess strong antibacterial, antifungal, and antiviral properties. Ranging from creamy white to dark brown in color, this gourmet honey (it can sell for more than $50 a pound) has been the centerpiece of Dr. Peter Molan's cutting-edge investigations at the Honey Research Unit at the University of Waikato since the 1980s.

While the results from Dr. Eddy of the University of Wisconsin Medical School described in the previous chapter show that even some types of common supermarket honey can help heal the most virulent diabetic foot ulcers, the Australian and New Zealand studies indicate that when it comes to treating wounds, it's best to choose a raw and unfiltered honey with proven antibacterial value.

At the present time, there is a lack of standardization of honey and honey dressings in terms of floral source, the quantity of honey needed for treatment, and the addition of other ingredients. Hopefully soon, pharmaceutical companies will recognize the value of producing standardized, microbe-free gamma-irradiated raw honey applications from a variety of floral sources that consumers and patients can buy in a drugstore and use easily at home.

Two Suggested Protocols

All serious and slow-healing wounds should be evaluated and treated under the supervision of a qualified health care practitioner, especially because the wounds may be the result of a more serious underlying problem such as diabetes. Yet the case that Dr. Eddy described in her article in which an elderly diabetic patient with amputated toes was treated by his family shows that you don't need to be a physician to successfully treat wounds with honey at home. Bee and honey expert Joe Traynor offered the following simple protocol in *Honey: The Gourmet Medicine*.

1. Abscesses, cavities, and depressions in the wound should be filled with honey before any dressing is applied.
2. Add one ounce of honey to a 4-inch square dressing pad and apply to the wound.
3. Apply a secondary dry dressing pad on top of the honey pad, and then use adhesive tape to hold both dressings in place.
4. Change dressings at least once a day (more frequently if much exudate is produced). Once the wound has stopped producing exudate, dressings can be changed once a week.[24]

Dr. Peter Molan offered the following recommendations for dressing wounds with honey, focusing on manuka honey that has proven antibacterial value.

1. Do not wait too long to start using honey on a wound.
2. Use only honey that has been selected for use in wound care.*
3. Use dressings that will hold sufficient honey in place on a wound to get a good therapeutic effect.
4. Ensure that honey is in full contact with the wound bed.

---

*Manuka honey for medicinal use: Apiban (Apimed: Cambridge, New Zealand), Woundcare 18+ (Comvita: Te Puke, New Zealand), and Medihoney (Capilano: Richlands, Queensland, Australia).

5. If a nonadherent dressing is used between the honey dressing and the wound bed, it must be sufficiently porous to allow the active components of the honey to diffuse through.

6. Ensure that honey dressings extend to cover any area of inflammation surrounding wounds.

7. Use a suitable secondary dressing to prevent leakage of honey.

8. Change the dressings frequently enough to prevent the honey [from] being washed away or excessively diluted by wound exudate.

9. When using honey to debride hard eschar [a scar formed especially after a burn], scoring and softening the eschar by soaking with saline will allow better penetration of the honey.[25]

Clearly there is a future for honey in wound treatment. Dr. Eddy and her coauthor, Mark D. Gideonsen, M.D., strongly agree with my assertion that "given honey's potential for improved outcomes, cost savings, and decreased antibiotic use and resistance, we advocate publicly funded randomized controlled trials to determine its efficacy. Meanwhile, we encourage others to consider topical honey for patients with refractory diabetic foot ulcers."[26]

Whether to treat foot ulcers due to diabetes, postoperative wounds, antibiotic-resistant skin infections, lesions related to cancer treatment, or for even simple cuts and abrasions, the scientific and clinical evidence shows that honey should be considered the first choice by physician and lay person alike. In the following chapter we'll learn how honey has gained worldwide renown for its ability to help heal a wide variety of burns.

8

HONEY FOR BURNS

*The slight regard at this time paid to the medicinal
virtues of honey is an instance of the neglect men show to
common objects, whatever their value.*

JOHN HILL, M.D. (1759)

Honey is a simple, inexpensive, and natural substance that has been used since ancient times by traditional and folk healers to treat burns. Like honey and wound healing in general, there has been little scientific research done on how honey can heal burns until recently.

What types of burns can honey treat? *Superficial burns* are limited to the epidermal or top layer of the skin. *Partial thickness burns* involve damage or problems with deeper structures of the skin, while the term *full thickness burns* indicates the destruction of all skin layers. Honey has been found to successfully treat the first two burn types.

In mainstream medical circles, there have been two standard treatments for burns. One involves a dressing that is a combination of paraffin-impregnated gauze, which is designed to prevent adherence to the burn, plus an absorbent layer of cotton and wool. The other is the use of silver sulfadiazine (SSD), which is prescribed primarily to fight infection. SSD has been used clinically since 1968 and is considered the "gold standard" for burn treatment by mainstream physicians throughout the world.

Problems in Treating Burns

Like wound healing in general, there are two major difficulties associated with treating burns. The first is the actual healing of the damaged tissue. The second is the danger of infection by microorganisms. For healing to occur, burn experts suggest that two things must happen.

1. Create environmental conditions within the wound that are favorable to the body's host repair mechanisms.
2. Make wound conditions unfavorable to the microorganisms.

How Honey Works to Help Heal Burns

As with wound care in general, honey provides a moist healing environment for burns. It also rapidly clears infection, deodorizes the burn area, and reduces inflammation, edema, and exudation. Honey also increases the rate of healing by stimulating the growth of new skin tissue and by reducing the need for skin grafts in the future. It also reduces the presence of scarring, which is a major problem among those who suffer from burn injuries.

Clinical Evidence: The India Trials

Some of the first peer-reviewed clinical trials of honey as a burn dressing were started in the early 1990s by Dr. M. Subrahmanyam of the Department of Surgery at Dr. Vaishampayan Memorial Medical College in Solapur (Maharashtra, India).

The first was a prospective randomized clinical study designed to compare honey-impregnated gauze to an amniotic-membrane dressing when applied to partial thickness burns. Dr. Subrahmanyam studied sixty-four patients with superficial burns: forty were treated with honey-impregnated gauze and twenty-four were treated with the amniotic membrane. He discovered that the burns treated with honey healed earlier than those treated with the amniotic membrane (an average of 9.4 days versus 17.5 days).

He also found that honey reduced burn scars more effectively. Residual scars were noted in 8 percent of patients treated with the honey-impregnated gauze and in 16.6 percent of cases treated with amniotic membrane.[1]

In another study—reported in the peer-reviewed journal *Burns* in 1998—Dr. Subrahmanyam compared the healing of burns with honey dressing and silver sulfadiazine (SSD). He created two groups of twenty-five randomly allocated patients. Of the twenty-five patients treated with honey, 84 percent showed satisfactory epithelialization by the seventh day and 100 percent by the twenty-first day. Among patients with wounds treated with silver sulfadiazine, epithelialization occurred by the seventh day in 72 percent of the twenty-five patients and in 84 percent of these patients by the twenty-first day.

When observed under a microscope, evidence of reparative activity was seen in 80 percent of wounds treated with the honey dressing by the seventh day with minimal inflammation, compared to 52 percent of the wounds treated with silver sulfadiazine. Reparative activity reached 100 percent by twenty-one days with the honey dressing and 84 percent with SSD.

Dr. Subrahmanyam concluded that honey not only controlled infection but also encouraged the growth of new tissue better than the SSD treatment. "Thus in honey dressed wounds, early subsidence of acute inflammatory changes, better control of infection and quicker wound healing was observed while in the SSD treated wounds sustained inflammatory reaction was noted even on epithelialization."[2]

Results of another Subrahmanyam study, reported in the *British Journal of Surgery,* suggest that honey possesses antibacterial properties that are superior to those of SSD. In this trial Dr. Subrahmanyam randomly assigned 104 patients with less than 40 percent total body surface area (TBSA) partial thickness burns to one of two groups. One group of fifty-two patients was treated with honey, and another group of fifty-two patients was treated with SSD cream. Biopsy specimens for culture and sensitivity determination were taken on admission, day seven, and day twenty-one of the study.

Findings revealed that honey was superior to SSD cream for preventing bacterial growth in the burn wound and for wound healing overall. In the fifty-two patients treated with honey, 91 percent of wounds were rendered sterile within seven days. In the fifty-two patients treated with SSD, only 7 percent showed control of infection within seven days. Healthy granulation tissue was observed earlier in patients treated with honey (mean 7.4 days versus 13.4 days). Of the wounds treated with honey, 87 percent healed within fifteen days as opposed to 10 percent in the control group treated with SSD cream.

Although Dr. Subrahmanyam's studies were not conducted in an outpatient setting—the total body surface area (TBSA) of the partial thickness burns was as high as 40 percent—these results suggest that honey may be a simple, inexpensive, alternative—and probably superior—dressing to use when treating minor burns.[3]

In an article appearing in the *Western Journal of Medicine,* a group of physicians from various medical departments at the University of California, Los Angeles (UCLA), evaluated all the published findings on silver sulfadiazine. They concluded that the traditional idea of SSD cream being the first-line treatment for minor burns is a "myth." In addition to the financial cost and its less than stellar ability to curb infection, they pointed out that SSD may place patients at increased risk for a variety of diseases, including neutropenia, erythema multiforme, crystalluria, and methemoglobinemia. They also found that honey is a better treatment by far due to superior performance, less cost, and lack of adverse side effects.[4]

Burns and *Pseudomonas aeruginosa*

Pseudomonas aeruginosa has been called the epitome of opportunistic human pathogens. This bacterium almost never infects uncompromised tissues, yet there is hardly any tissue that it cannot infect if the body's natural defenses are compromised in any way.

While *Pseudomonas* is found in perhaps 4 percent of infected wounds, it is far more common among burn patients, especially when the burns are extensive. If left untreated, *Pseudomonas* can cause a variety of diseases, including urinary tract infections, respiratory system infections, soft tissue infections, bone and joint infections, gastrointestinal infections, and a variety of systemic infections. *Pseudomonas* is notoriously resistant to antimicrobial therapy.

Honey versus *Pseudomonas*

In 1998 Dr. Rose Cooper of the School of Microbiological Sciences at the University of Wales Institute and Dr. Peter Molan of the Department of Biological Sciences at the University of Waikato undertook a pioneer laboratory study to determine the effectiveness of the antibacterial properties of honey against *Pseudomonas*. They isolated *Pseudomonas* from twenty infected wounds, and the cultures were inoculated with various concentrations of pasture honey and manuka honey.

They calculated that the concentration of honey required to completely inhibit *Pseudomonas* growth averaged 7.1 percent for the pasture honey (with a range of 5.8 to 9.0 percent), and that of manuka honey was 6.9 percent (with a range of 5.5 to 8.7 percent). They also discovered that honey could be diluted up to ten times by wound exudate and still be effective in inhibiting *Pseudomonas* growth.[5]

Several years later Cooper and Molan again focused their research on burns infected with this bacterium. They tested the sensitivity of seventeen strains of *Pseudomonas aeruginosa* isolated from infected burns to both pasture honey and manuka honey with median levels of antibacterial activity.

As in their earlier study described above, all of the strains of *Pseudomonas aeruginosa* were completely inhibited by both honeys at a 10 percent concentration, and both honeys maintained their antibacterial activity even when diluted more than tenfold. After noting that honey was found to manage infections from burns better than silver sulfadiazine and also reduces scarring from burns, the researchers concluded:

> These beneficial effects of honey and its lack of adverse effects on wounds, considered along with the findings from the present study, indicate that honey with standardized antibacterial activity has the potential to be a very useful treatment option for burns infected or at risk for infection with *Pseudomonas aeruginosa*.[6]

Two more articles were recently published in scientific journals that substantiated Cooper and Molan's earlier results. In one study Dr. Jenny

M. Wilkinson and Heather M. A. Cavanagh of the School of Biomedical Sciences at Charles Sturt University in Australia evaluated the activity of thirteen honeys, including three commercial antibacterial honeys, against *Escherichia coli* and *Pseudomonas aeruginosa*. Antibacterial activity of the honeys was assayed using standard well-diffusion methods. All the honeys, along with an artificial honey, were tested at four concentrations (10 percent, 5 percent, 2.5 percent, and 1 percent) against *E. coli* and *P. aeruginosa,* and zones of inhibition were measured.

All honeys tested had an inhibitory effect on the growth of *E. coli* and *P. aeruginosa,* with one honey still having activity against *E. coli* and three having activity against *P. aeruginosa* at a concentration of 2.5 percent. No honey was active at 1 percent concentration.

They found that *E. coli* was more susceptible to inhibition by the honeys used in this study than was *P. aeruginosa*. The authors concluded: "In this study we have demonstrated that several honeys, in addition to commercial antibacterial honeys, can inhibit *E. coli* and *P. aeruginosa* and may have potential as therapeutic honeys."[7]

An article by Dr. L. Boukraa and Dr. A. Niar at the Ibn Khaldoun University of Tiaret in Algeria published in the December 2007 issue of the *Journal of Medicinal Food* compared the antibacterial activity of six varieties of honey from different regions in Algeria against *Pseudomonas aeruginosa*. Four varieties originated from northern Algeria, and two from the Sahara. Three types of media were used.

On nutrient agar, the minimum inhibitory concentration (MIC) of the four northern varieties ranged between 30 percent and 31 percent. The MIC of the Sahara varieties was 11 percent and 14 percent. On King A agar, the MIC of the four northern varieties ranged from 25 percent to 31 percent, whereas the MIC of the two varieties of Sahara honey was 12 percent and 15 percent. On nutrient broth, the MIC of the northern varieties ranged from 10 percent to 21 percent, whereas the MIC of the two varieties of Sahara honey was 9 percent.

Noting that the botanic flora of the Algerian Sahara is historically known for its wide variety of medicinal uses, the higher potency of the Sahara honey is most probably due to antibacterial substances in the plant nectars from that region. The researchers concluded: "These findings suggest that Sahara honey could be used for managing wounds and burns, which are mostly infected by *P. aeruginosa*."[8]

Toward the Future

Treating burns with honey was standard practice in times past but went out of fashion with the development of antibiotics. Yet as the evidence shows, honey is a powerful antibacterial agent that is effective against several major types of burns. Free from adverse side effects, honey kills dangerous bacteria while it encourages the growth of healthy tissue. It also reduces the potential for scarring, a major problem with burns. The development of new honey-based antiseptic creams and sterile dressings also makes burn treatment easier and more effective than even ten years ago.

With the growing problem of antibiotic-resistant bacteria among burn patients in hospitals today, doctors may do well to take a second look at the potential of honey as a broad-spectrum antibacterial agent that is inexpensive, effective, and free from the adverse side effects so common with modern antibiotics.

9

HONEY AND
INTERNAL DISORDERS

*The secret of my health is applying honey inside and oil
outside.*

DEMOCRITUS

The Greek philosopher Democritus (ca. 460–ca. 370 BCE) was the co-originator of the belief that all matter is made up of various imperishable, indivisible elements that he called *atoma,* or "indivisible units," from which we get the English word atom. He was also known as the "laughing philosopher" because he seemed to have achieved happiness through inner tranquillity.

According to the compiler and writer Stobaeus, Democritus counseled reason and balance when dealing with issues of lifestyle and health. His health advice was lent credibility by the fact that Democritus lived to be a very old man. Although some claim that he lived a mere ninety years, the astronomer and mathematician Hipparchus assures us that Democritus died at the age of 109. When asked the secret of his extreme longevity, Democritus answered that he anointed his body with olive oil and ate honey daily.

In the previous chapters I discussed how honey is an ideal healer for treating various types of wounds and burns. Honey not only has potent antibacterial and anti-inflammatory effects when applied to wounds, but it can also help reduce both swelling and pain that is not just a result of clearing infection and debriding the wound.

Although honey has been taken internally as a folk remedy since even before the time of Democritus, very little scientific research has documented its healthful effects in the prevention and cure of various diseases during the past sixty years or so. While clearly more research needs to be done—especially double-blind human studies—a sampling of available scientific data reveals a wide range of honey's therapeutic applications.

Honey and Cough

Although honey has been used by traditional and folk healers to treat colds and coughs for thousands of years, it has only recently been cited by the World Health Organization as a potential treatment for these ailments.[1]

In its report on the treatment of upper respiratory tract infections, the WHO cites honey as a demulcent—a substance that relieves throat irritation—that is cheap, popular, and safe for young children. In addition to the demulcent effect, honey has antioxidant properties and increases cytokine release, which may explain its antimicrobial effects.

In 2007 a group of researchers from the Pennsylvania State University published the results of a survey showing that a single nighttime dose of buckwheat honey was more effective than the popular medication dextromethorphan (DM) on both nocturnal cough and sleep difficulty associated with childhood upper respiratory tract infections. One hundred and five children aged two to eighteen years with upper respiratory tract infections, nocturnal symptoms, and illness duration of seven days or less were involved in the study, which focused on the child's parents filling out a questionnaire. After a single dose of buckwheat honey, honey-flavored DM, or no treatment at all was administered thirty minutes before bedtime, the frequency, severity, and discomfort of cough were evaluated as well as the child's ability to sleep through the night.

The researchers found "significant differences in symptom improvement" among treatment groups, with honey consistently scoring the best and no treatment scoring the worst. In paired comparisons, honey was "significantly superior" to "no treatment" for cough frequency. It also ranked better when cough severity, bothersome nature of cough, and child/parent sleep quality were considered. By contrast, DM did not score better than "no treatment" for dealing with cough frequency or any other of the related cough/sleep problems. Comparison of honey with DM revealed no significant differences. However, unlike honey—which is totally safe to use—dextromethorphan has been associated with a variety of serious adverse side effects, even at recommended doses. In addition, both pre-teens and teenagers often abuse DM as a recreational drug.

In their article published in the December 3, 2007, issue of the peer-reviewed *Archives of Pediatric and Adolescent Medicine,* the researchers concluded:

> In a comparison of honey, DM, and no treatment, parents rated honey most favorably for symptomatic relief of their child's nocturnal cough and sleep difficulty due to upper respiratory tract infection. Honey may be a preferable treatment for the cough and sleep difficulty associated with childhood upper respiratory tract infection.[2]

Honey and Intestinal Disorders

The ancient Assyrians, Greeks, Egyptians, and Chinese used honey to not only heal skin-related wounds but also to cure stomach and intestinal complaints. Hippocrates—often referred to as "The Father of Medicine"—recommended eating honey to heal gastritis. In recent times, consuming honey to treat intestinal tract diseases has been documented in medical literature since 1949, including gastrointestinal infections like gastritis, duodenitis, and gastric ulcer caused by bacteria and rotovirus.[3] Most of the studies suggested that healing was brought about primarily through honey's antibacterial activity.

I mentioned earlier that gastrointestinal microflora is recognized as an important factor in intestinal and overall health. Increasing the populations of *Bifidobacterium* and other "healthy bacteria" in the intestines has been found to be important in both aiding digestion and helping to protect the body from harmful pathogens.[4]

The results of a study done at Michigan State University and reported in the *Journal of Food Protection* revealed that honey enhanced the growth of human *Bifidobacterium* in the intestine, probably due to the oligosaccharides that are present in honey at levels of 4 to 5 percent.[5]

The human intestine is normally coated with mucus, which is a viscid and slippery secretion rich in mucoproteins. It is produced by mucous membranes that the secretions moisten and protect. In order for gastrointestinal infection to take place, bacteria must be able to both adhere to and colonize this delicate mucosal surface. Clinicians have proposed that blocking the attachment of bacteria to the intestinal epithelium (the membranous tissue that covers the surface of the intestine) is a potential strategy for disease prevention.

Salmonella

Salmonella is a bacterium that causes typhoid fever, paratyphoid fever, and food-borne illness. Most persons infected with *Salmonella* develop diarrhea, fever, and abdominal cramps from twelve to seventy-two hours after infection. Symptoms usually last from four to seven days, and most persons recover without treatment. However, in some persons the diarrhea may be so severe that the patient needs to be hospitalized. In severe cases, the infection may spread from the intestines to the bloodstream and then to other body sites. It can cause death unless the person is treated promptly with antibiotics. The elderly, infants, and those with impaired immune systems are more likely to have a severe illness than others.

A pioneer in vitro study was carried out in 2003 by a team of microbiologists and immunologists from the College of Medicine and Health Sciences at Sultan Qaboos University in Oman. The researchers' goal was to determine the antimicrobial properties of honey and whether honey can prevent the bacteria *Salmonella enteritis* from adhering to the intestinal wall.

Using cultures of *S. enteritis* from a British laboratory and four different types of unadulterated Omani honey, the researchers evaluated the antibacterial value of honey on the epithelial cells of the small intestines of mice. While the *Salmonella* bacteria readily adhered to and colonized untreated cells, they could not adhere to cells treated with honey, even at dilutions of up to 1:8. Although the researchers couldn't explain the reasons for this scientifically, three opinions were presented.

1. Nonspecific mechanical inhibition may have occurred through the coating of the bacteria by the honey.
2. Some of the phytochemicals found in honey may have altered the electrostatic charge that allows bacteria to adhere to the intestinal wall.
3. The honey simply kills the bacteria outright.[6]

Though research on humans needs to be done, this groundbreaking research reveals how honey can be a powerful preventive medicine in regions where *Salmonella* infection is prevalent.

Infantile Gastroenteritis

Infantile gastroenteritis is a common viral infection that affects infants and children. Also known as gastric flu and stomach flu (although it's unrelated to influenza), this disease consists of inflammation of the gastrointestinal tract, involving both the stomach and the small intestine, resulting in acute diarrhea. Diarrhea causes dehydration and is a common cause of death among young children, especially in the developing countries of the world.

Viral infections are the main cause of gastroenteritis in infants and children and at least half of the cases result from consuming infected food or unsafe water: by the age of five nearly every child will have experienced at least one episode of rotavirus gastroenteritis. Worldwide, inadequate treatment of gastroenteritis kills an estimated five to eight million people per year, especially in developing countries.

A group of pediatricians from the Faculty of Medicine at the University of Natal in South Africa undertook a study using honey in an oral rehydration solution in infants and children with gastroenteritis at the

R. K. Khan Hospital in Durban. One hundred and sixty infants and children aged eight days to eleven years took part in the study. The children were divided into two groups: one group (eighty-nine patients) received routine management for diarrhea, which included oral fluids alone and/or intravenous fluids containing glucose and electrolytes. The second group (eighty patients) was given a drink containing 50 ml of honey per liter, with the electrolyte content equal to the drink given to group one.

The results, which were reported in the *British Medical Journal*, showed that honey shortens the duration of diarrhea in patients with bacterial gastroenteritis caused by organisms like *Salmonella*, *Shigella*, and *E. coli*. The researchers also found that honey does not prolong the duration of nonbacterial diarrhea. Pointing out that honey was safe, nonallergenic, and readily available in most communities, they concluded that honey "may safely be used as a substitute for glucose in an oral rehydration solution containing electrolytes."[7]

Dyspepsia and Stomach Ulcers

Honey has long been a traditional folk remedy to treat dyspepsia, a common health complaint that involves chronic or recurrent pain or discomfort centered in the upper abdomen.

The finding that *Helicobacter pylori* is probably the cause of many cases of dyspepsia has raised the possibility that the therapeutic action of honey may be due to its antibacterial properties. Consequently, a team of researchers from the Department of Biological Sciences at the University of Waikato in Hamilton, New Zealand, tested the sensitivity of *Helicobacter pylori* to honey using isolates from biopsies of gastric ulcers.

It was found that all five isolates tested were killed by a 20 percent (v/v) solution of manuka honey in an agar well-diffusion assay. However, none showed sensitivity to a 40 percent solution of a honey in which the antibacterial activity was due primarily to its content of hydrogen peroxide.

Assessment of the MIC by inclusion of manuka honey in the agar showed that all seven isolates of *Helicobacter* tested had visible growth over the incubation period of seventy-two hours prevented completely by the presence of 5 percent of manuka honey.[8]

A study undertaken twelve years later by researchers at the Department of Microbiology and Immunology, College of Medicine and Health Sciences at Sultan Qaboos University, sought to assess the antibacterial potential of eight types of honey sold in the city of Muscat (the capital and largest city of Oman) on isolates of *Helicobacter pylori*. They also wanted to find if there was a synergistic effect between honey and two traditional therapies—clarithromycin and amoxicillin—for *H. pylori* gastritis and duodenal ulcer.

The researchers found that all honey samples inhibited growth of *H. pylori* at no dilution, but there are different zones of inhibition at 1:2 to 1:8 dilutions. Overall, Black Forest honey was found to have the highest antibacterial activity, followed by Langnese brand honey, a premium German honey often available at gourmet food stores. They observed neither synergy nor antagonism between honey and clarithromycin or honey and amoxicillin using *H. pylori* as a test organism.[9]

Cystic Fibrosis

Cystic fibrosis (CF), or mucoviscoidosis, is a hereditary disease that affects mainly the lungs and digestive system, causing progressive disability. *Burkholderia cepacia* is an opportunistic pathogen that causes lung infections in patients suffering from cystic fibrosis. It is often very resistant to antibiotics and notoriously difficult to treat.

Dr. Rose Cooper and her colleagues at the School of Applied Sciences at the University of Wales Institute isolated twenty strains of antibiotic-resistant *Burkholderia cepacia* from the sputum of cystic fibrosis patients. Assessing the strains of the bacteria with an agar-dilution method, the researchers found that all of them were killed by both UMF-rated Manuka and mixed pasture honey in concentrations below 6 percent. They concluded that honey—perhaps administered in the form of aerosols—might have a potential role in the clinical management of *Burkholderia cepacia* infections.

However, the researchers cautioned that manuka honey was a preferable treatment for CF patients who were also infected with *Pseudomonas aeruginosa,* because hydrogen peroxide–generating honey could induce conversion of nonmucoid strains of the virus to more virulent forms.[10]

Hemorrhoids

New York– and Dubai-based physician Noori Al-Waili and his colleagues undertook a prospective pilot study to evaluate the therapeutic effect of topical application of a mixture of honey, olive oil, and beeswax on patients with anal fissure or hemorrhoids.

They selected fifteen patients—thirteen males and two females—with a median age of forty-five years (with a range of twenty-eight to seventy), who were diagnosed with either anal fissure (five patients) or first- to third-degree hemorrhoids (four with first degree, four with second degree, and two with third degree). They were treated with a twelve-hour application of a natural mixture containing honey, olive oil, and beeswax in ratio of 1:1:1(v/v/v).

Bleeding, itching, edema, and erythema were measured using the following scoring method: 0 = none, 1 = mild, 2 = moderate, 3 = severe, and 4 = very severe. The pain score was checked using a visual analog scale with a minimum of 0 and a maximum of 10.

Efficacy of treatment was assessed by comparing the symptoms' score before and after treatment at weekly intervals for a maximum of four weeks. The patients were observed for evidence of adverse effects such as the appearance of new signs and symptoms, or worsening of the existing symptoms.

Dr. Al-Waili and his team found that the honey mixture significantly reduced bleeding and relieved itching in patients with hemorrhoids. Patients with anal fissure showed significant reduction in pain, bleeding, and itching after the treatment. No side effects were reported. They concluded: "A mixture of honey, olive oil, and beeswax is safe and clinically effective in the treatment of hemorrhoids and anal fissure, which paves the way for further randomized double-blind studies."[11]

Honey: A Possible Cure for Yeast Infection?

Members of the Department of Microbiology at Erciyes University in Kayseri, Turkey, carried out an in vitro study on the antifungal activity of Turkish honey against both *Candida* and *Trichosporon*.

The researchers evaluated honey samples from various floral sources for their ability to inhibit the growth of forty yeast strains, including *Candida albicans, C. krusei, C. glabrata,* and *Trichosporon* spp. Fluconazole-resistant yeast strains were also examined for their susceptibility to honey. Fluconazole is used to treat fungal infections, including yeast infections of the vagina, mouth, throat, esophagus, and urinary tract.

The researchers found that all of the yeast strains tested were inhibited by honeys in this study. Broth microdilution assay revealed that inhibition of growth depends on the type and concentration of honey as well as the test pathogen. Little or no antifungal activity was seen at honey concentrations of less than 2 percent. They also found that rhododendron and multifloral honeys have generally more of an inhibitory effect than eucalyptus and orange honey varieties. Writing in the December 2008 issue of *Medical Mycology,* the authors concluded: "This study demonstrated that, in vitro, these honeys had antifungal activity at the high concentration of 80% (v/v) in these fluconazole-resistant strains. Further studies are now required to demonstrate if this antifungal activity has any clinical application."[12]

10

HONEY IN ORAL
HEALTH AND
OPHTHALMOLOGY

*The use of honey on human beings over a period of more
than 4,000 years, with no adverse effects coming to light,
is evidence of its effectiveness as a healing agent.*

PETER C. MOLAN, PROFESSOR OF BIOLOGICAL SCIENCES
AND DIRECTOR OF THE HONEY RESEARCH UNIT,
UNIVERSITY OF WAIKATO, NEW ZEALAND

The subject of honey and oral health is a controversial one. On one level,
honey—like other sugars—causes dental cavities. It has been said that the
honey bear is the only animal found in nature with a problem with tooth
decay.

A 2005 study at the University of Rochester Medical Center in New
York about the cavity-causing potentials of different foods given to infants
and toddlers placed honey among the most cavity-promoting of sweeteners, ranking it just behind soda beverages and table sugar (sucrose).
Researchers assigned each liquid substance an arbitrary value of 1 and
scored the cariogenicity (cavity-producing ability) of each substance based
on the number and severity of lesions that developed on the rats' teeth

bloodstream and eventually to the heart, causing infection and possible heart attack.[3]

While regular brushing and careful dental flossing are considered the best ways to fight periodontal disease, there are several promising honey-related applications as well. The same gelled-honey dressing as discussed for oral surgical wounds but formulated in softer form—addition to specially formulated honey candies—can also be applied to periodontal and other mouth infections. Dr. Molan wrote: "Its antibacterial activity would provide anti-infective therapy in periodontal disease by removing the etiological factor and the anti-inflammatory activity would block the direct cause of the erosion of the connective tissues and bone."[4] He added: "Another beneficial feature of using honey to treat periodontal disease would be its well-established stimulation of growth of granulation tissue and epithelial cells, which would aid in repair of the damage done by infecting bacteria and by the inflammatory response to free radicals."[5]

Honey and Gingivitis

Gingivitis is a common oral-health problem involving inflammation of the gums. It is caused by bacterial biofilms (also called plaque) that adhere to tooth surfaces. Most people have suffered from gingivitis from time to time, diagnosed by one or more of the following symptoms: swollen gums, mouth sores, bright-red or purple gums, shiny gums, gums that don't hurt except when pressure is applied, gums that bleed easily even with gentle brushing and especially when flossing, itching gums, and receding gum line.

A joint pilot study carried out by researchers in the School of Dentistry in Dunedin, New Zealand, and the Honey Research Unit at the University of Waikato found that manuka honey with an activity rated UMF 15 could be used clinically to reduce dental plaque and clinical levels of gingivitis.

Thirty male and female volunteers (with an average age of forty-nine) were selected for the randomized trial. Half were given a special manuka "honey leather" product, and the other half received sugarless chewing gum. They were to chew the honey leather or gum for ten minutes three times a day after each meal for twenty-one days. Plaque and gum bleeding were recorded before and after the trial.

The researchers found that there were "highly significant" reductions in dental plaque (0.99 reduced to 0.65) in the manuka group, whereas plaque reduction in the control group was "slight." Gingivitis in the group given manuka honey fell by 48 percent, while that of the controls fell 17 percent. The researchers believe that the antibacterial properties of the honey might have been the major reason why gum bleeding was reduced so markedly. While acknowledging the need for a much larger clinical trial, they concluded: "These results suggest that there may be a potential therapeutic role for manuka honey confectionery in the treatment of gingivitis and periodontal disease."[6]

Honey and Root Canal Treatment?

From August through November 2001, Dr. M. B. Sobhi and Dr. M. A. Manzoor from the Operative Dentistry Department at the Armed Forces Institutes of Dentistry in Rawalpindi, Pakistan, compared the efficacy of camphorated paramonochlorophenol to a mixture of honey and mustard oil as a root canal medicine.

They collected ninety samples of infected contents from decayed teeth in root canal patients from the Operative Dentistry Department of the Armed Forces Institute of Dentistry. Organisms were identified, and isolates were preserved and refrigerated for the experiments. They also prepared the medicines in comparable dilutions. The minimum inhibitory concentration of both medicaments was determined by susceptibility testing against already preserved isolates. The researchers found that both the mixture of honey and mustard oil and the camphorated paramonochlorophenol demonstrated antibacterial activity. Although the concentration of the honey and mustard oil was greater, the researchers concluded that it was nevertheless "[an] effective, viable alternate endodontic medicament."[7]

Honey: Good for the Eyes?

Although there is evidence that the ancient Egyptians used honey to treat eye diseases, the Greek philosopher Aristotle is credited with being among the first to record medicinal use of honey for the eyes as far back as 350 BCE. In section 627a of his tome *Historia Animalium,* he wrote: "White honey . . . is good as a salve for sore eyes." Honey was also widely used in India to treat eye diseases and has been used by traditional healers in Mali to prevent scarring of the cornea in cases of measles.[8] In chapter 4 I cited references from the Talmud about the healing effects of honey on the eyes ("Honey enlightens the eyes of man"), and there is also evidence that honey was used by the medieval English to treat eye diseases.[9]

Like the treatment of wounds and burns described earlier, honey's applications in ophthalmology—a branch of medical science dealing with the structure, functions, and diseases of the eye—are primarily anti-inflammatory, antibacterial, and antifungal. One of the earliest ophthalmology-related reports was published in the Soviet Union in 1953. It described using honey in place of petroleum jelly in a 3 percent sulfidine eye ointment to treat keratitis, a disease in which the cornea of the eye is inflamed. It also reported positive results with the honey ointment for twenty-eight patients suffering from a variety of eye problems, including syphilitic keratitis, corneal ulcers, injuries to the cornea, and lime burns to the cornea.[10]

A later study, reported by a team of Soviet researchers in 1984, documented the use of honey to cure a variety of eye diseases, including opaque spots appearing in the cornea as a result of herpes, chemical and thermal burns to the eye, and conjunctivitis.[11]

In 1988, Dr. M. H. Emarah reported anecdotal evidence of successful eye treatments with honey in the *Bulletin of Islamic Medicine.* Patients at an Egyptian clinic were given topical applications of honey two to three times daily. Conditions treated included chronic nonspecific conjunctivitis and consistent inflammation of the eyelids, a condition known as blepharitis.[12]

In his three-part article in the journal *Bee World* about honey in medicine, Dr. Peter Molan cited the work of Dr. M. C. Sarma, an ophthalmic surgeon at the Rangaraya Medical College in India. Dr. Sarma is successfully treating bacterial corneal ulcers with honey, as well as inflammation of the eyelids, catarrhal conjunctivitis, and keratitis.[13]

Dr. Ahmad M. Mansour and colleagues at the Department of Ophthalmology at the American University of Beirut undertook a prospective study with twenty-four patients suffering from bullous keratopathy, a major complication of cataract surgery. Plastic surgery—particularly corneal grafting—is considered the most effective therapy for this disease. One drop of honey was applied to the cornea three to four times daily. Although patients experienced a stinging sensation at first, discomfort became minimal after repeated use. Improvement in visual acuity and corneal clearing lasted for about an hour after the honey applications. The researchers were impressed with the results. In a letter appearing in *Acta Ophthalmologica Scandinavica* in 2004, they conclude: "Given its advantages in terms of its antimicrobial, antioxidant, anti-inflammatory and hygroscopic [readily taking up and retaining moisture] properties, further evaluation of the long term effects of honey on bullous keratopathy is warranted."[14]

Another study about honey to treat eye diseases was published in *Georgian Medical News* in 2007. Aware of the role of antioxidants in protecting the body from the formation of free radicals, a team of physicians from the country of Georgia developed honey-based eye drops with high antioxidant activity and called the product Davicoli. They measured the ocular effects of the eye drops in a placebo-controlled double-blind study involving forty-four mice, forty-four rats, forty sea pigs, and twenty chinchillas. Their findings revealed that the eye drops not only reduced inflammation but were also safe and nontoxic.[15]

The potential for honey eye drops and salves to help treat a variety of eye conditions is promising indeed. While anecdotal evidence and animal experiments may be of value, the most useful evidence will come from placebo-controlled double-blind studies with human subjects. Like the honey-based creams, salves, and bandages to treat wounds and burns described in the previous chapters, the development of products to treat eye diseases will not lag too far behind.

11

HONEY: SAFE FOR INFANTS? SAFE FOR DIABETICS?

*Infants younger than 12 months are at risk of infant
botulism from eating honey.*

JAY HOECKER, M.D.

Honey has long been considered a safe and healthy food for children and adults. Although it has been given to infants as both food and medicine since ancient Egyptian times, doctors like Jay Hoecker, a pediatrician at the Mayo Clinic, recommend that honey not be given to infants under one year of age.

Why is this? Infants are especially vulnerable to botulism, which is caused by spores of the bacterium *Clostridium botulinum*. They do not affect children and adults. Yet because the gastrointestinal tract of infants is not fully developed—they do not yet have the intestinal microflora that allow them to ingest the *C. botulinum* spores without harm—the spores can germinate and grow in the intestinal tract and produce the deadly disease.

Clostridium botulinum is widely found in nature. Scientists have detected it in the soil, in the air, and in house dust, which can contaminate toys, feeding bottles, pacifiers, and baby's hands. It is also found in fresh and processed meats, corn syrup, fruits, and vegetables.

Clostridium botulinum spores have also been found in a tiny number of honey samples. It is very difficult to remove these spores without destroying the honey itself. Although the chances of an infant coming down with botulism from honey is remote, the United States Centers for Disease Prevention and Control, the American Academy of Pediatrics, and the National Honey Board all advise that honey should not be fed to infants under one year of age.

A Difference of Opinion

Not all scientists agree with this recommendation. In chapter 9 I cited a clinical trial dealing with honey's ability to treat infantile gastroenteritis. In this study, a group of pediatricians from the Faculty of Medicine at the University of Natal in South Africa treated children as young as eight days of age with honey.

Mamdouh AbdulRhman, M.D., and Nermeen Tayseer, M.D. (Dr. AbdulRhaman is a professor of pediatrics and Dr. Tayseer is a lecturer in clinical pathology at Ain Shams University in Cairo), undertook a study at Al Khafji National Hospital in Saudi Arabia from 1998 to 2002. Their study included laboratory testing, a patient survey, and examination of hospital records regarding honey and infant botulism. They concluded that the recommendation that honey should not be given to infants should be reevaluated.

The researchers examined a total of 221 honey samples for the presence of *C. botulinum* spores by direct gram-stained films and cultures for forty-eight hours under strict anaerobic conditions. One hundred and fifteen honey samples were from the Kingdom of Saudi Arabia: seventy of these were of commercial origin, whereas forty-five were from local producers. The remaining 106 honey samples were from the United States, Germany, Switzerland, China, Australia, Pakistan, Turkey, Egypt, Yemen, Sudan, Syria, and Iran. *Clostridium* spores were not detected in any of the honey samples.

In addition, questions were posed directly to 719 mothers who were randomly chosen from the hospital's files. They were asked how many children were given honey before the age of one year, at what age honey was first given, and whether there was any mortality or significant illness that could be attributed to infant botulism among those children.

The questionnaire revealed that 545 out of 719 mothers (75.8 percent) fed honey to their infants (1,525 infants) at least once before the age of one year without mortality or significant illness that could be attributed to botulism. None of those infants developed manifestations suggestive of botulism, and none developed serious respiratory illness. A total of 378 mothers (69 percent) used honey as a food and as a medicine that they felt not only helped their children get better but also led to less frequent doctor visits. Thirty-one percent (167) of the mothers fed honey to their infants as food only. Of the 1,525 infants given honey, the majority (56.2 percent) were more than six months of age while just 57 (3.7 percent) of the infants were twenty-eight days of age or younger.

The researchers also found that no case of infant botulism was reported between 1995 and 2002 in the three hospitals of Al Khafji or in the local health office.[1]

Recommendations

The decision to give honey to an infant is a difficult one. While medical-grade UMF-rated Manuka honey that has been gamma irradiated to kill *Clostridium* spores would be a possible solution to this problem, this type of honey is not easy to obtain.

Mothers need to make the decision as to whether giving honey to their baby is worth the risk or if feeding honey should simply be delayed until it can produce no health problems.

Is Honey Safe for Diabetics?

According to the American Diabetes Association, diabetes is a disease in which the body does not produce or properly use insulin. Insulin is a hormone that is needed to convert sugar, starches, and other food into energy for daily life. While the cause of diabetes is a mystery, both genetic and environmental factors—such as obesity and lack of exercise—appear to play roles.

There are two major types of diabetes:

- Type-1 diabetes results from the body's failure to produce insulin, the hormone that "unlocks" the cells of the body, allowing glucose to enter and fuel them. It is estimated that 5 to 10 percent of Americans who are diagnosed with diabetes have this type.
- Type-2 diabetes results from insulin resistance (a condition in which the body fails to properly use insulin) combined with relative insulin deficiency. Most Americans who are diagnosed with diabetes have type-2 diabetes.[2]

Honey and the Glycemic Index

The glycemic index (GI) is a ranking system for carbohydrates based on their effect on blood glucose levels. It compares available carbohydrates in individual foods and provides a specific glycemia index that occurs two hours after the food is consumed.

Carbohydrates that break down rapidly during digestion have the highest glycemic indices, while those that break down slowly, releasing glucose gradually into the blood stream, have a low glycemic index. A lower glycemic response is often thought to equate to a lower insulin demand, better long-term blood glucose control, and a reduction in blood lipids.

Two of the foods with the highest GI indices are sugars and highly refined carbohydrates. The average American consumes between two and three pounds of sugar each week, mostly in the form of sucrose (table sugar), dextrose (corn sugar), and high-fructose corn syrup. These are found in abundance in many of the prepared foods we eat every day, including bread, breakfast cereal, mayonnaise, peanut butter, ketchup, spaghetti sauce, and a plethora of microwave and ready-to-serve meals. We also eat large amounts of white flour products, including bread, rolls, pastry, rice, pasta, and cereals, which all have high glycemic index levels.

- High glycemic foods range from 64 to 100 on the glycemic index and include raisins, breakfast cereals, white bread, and table sugar. Glucose has the highest level of 100.

- Medium glycemic foods range from 41 to 57 on the glycemic index and include apple juice, rice, sweet potatoes, bananas, and oranges.
- Low glycemic foods score from 25 to 36 on the glycemic index and include beans and pulses, apples, pears, and skim milk.

Depending on the type, honey generally has a glycemic index of between 35 (Romanian locust honey) and 87 (unspecified Canadian honey). Yet in spite of the somewhat higher glycemic index than even table sugar, honey has been able to actually contribute to low increases in glucose levels, even among diabetics.

The Dubai Studies

Two unusual broad-spectrum studies about honey and glucose levels were carried out by Dr. Noori Al-Waili at the Dubai Specialized Medical Center, Islamic Establishment for Education, in Dubai, United Arab Emirates.

The first study was designed to determine the safety and effectiveness of intrapulmonary administration (by inhalation) of a 60 percent honey solution and a 10 percent dextrose or distilled water solution on blood sugar, plasma insulin and C-peptide, blood pressure, heart rate, and peaked expiratory flow rate (PEFR) in normal and diabetic subjects. Plasma C-peptide is an amino acid that may reflect pancreatic insulin secretion more reliably than the level of insulin itself. Twenty-four healthy participants along with sixteen patients diagnosed with type-2 diabetes mellitus and six patients with hypertension participated in the study.

Results showed that in normal subjects, distilled water caused a mild elevation in blood glucose levels, mild lowering of plasma insulin, and significant reduction of plasma C-peptide. A 10 percent dextrose inhalation caused mild reduction of plasma insulin and C-peptide and unremarkable changes in blood glucose levels. Dr. Al-Waili found no significant changes in blood pressure, heart rate, or PEFR after either distilled water or the 10 percent dextrose inhalation.

By contrast, he found that the honey inhalation caused lowering of blood glucose level and an elevation of plasma insulin and C-peptide, a mild reduction of blood pressure, and up to a 16 percent increase in PEFR. In addition, the honey inhalation significantly reduced random blood glucose levels approximately 25 percent. He also found that the intensity of hyperglycemia was significantly lowered in the glucose tolerance test when patients received the honey inhalation.

Among patients with high blood pressure, he found that their systolic and diastolic blood pressure was reduced by honey inhalation, with "significant" changes obtained at 60 and 120 minutes after inhalation. Dr. Al-Waili concluded: "The results demonstrated that honey inhalation was safe and effective in reducing blood glucose level in normal and diabetic subjects, it could improve glucose tolerance test, elevate plasma insulin and C-peptide and PEFR, and reduce elevated blood pressure in hypertensive patients."[3]

His second broad-spectrum study involved fifty-three patients. It focused on comparing the effects of dextrose solution and honey solution on plasma glucose level (PGL), plasma insulin, and plasma C-peptide. He then compared solutions made with honey, dextrose alone, or dextrose and fructose on levels of blood cholesterol and triglycerides. Finally, Dr. Al-Waili analyzed the effects of a honey solution on levels of PGL, blood lipids, C-reactive protein (CRP), homocysteine (an amino acid; high levels have been linked to heart disease), triglycerides, and cholesterol.

While further random studies utilizing a larger number of subjects could produce more definitive results regarding diabetes, Dr. Al-Waili's findings show the medicinal value of honey for people at risk for diabetes, heart disease, and circulatory problems. He concluded: "Honey reduces blood lipids, homocysteine, and CRP in normal and hyperlipidemic subjects. Honey compared with dextrose and sucrose caused lower elevation of PGL in diabetics."[4]

The India Study

In 2006 a team of researchers from the School of Studies in Zoology at Jiwaji University in India compared the relative tolerance to honey and glucose among adults with impaired glucose tolerance or mild diabetes.

Thirty thirty-five- to sixty-year-old individuals with a proven parental (mother or father) history of type-2 diabetes mellitus were simultaneously given an oral glucose tolerance test (GTT) and a honey tolerance test (HTT). Glucose tolerance was found to be impaired in twenty-four subjects, while six of the subjects were diagnosed as mildly diabetic.

All subjects with impaired glucose tolerance exhibited significantly lower plasma glucose concentrations after consumption of honey at all time points of the honey tolerance test in comparison to the glucose tolerance test. The plasma glucose levels in response to honey peaked at thirty to sixty minutes and showed a rapid decline as compared to that of glucose. The researchers noted that the high degree of tolerance to honey was recorded in subjects with diabetes as well, indicating a lower glycemic index for honey.

Although the researchers didn't advocate heavy honey consumption among diabetics, they concluded: ". . . honey may prove to be a valuable sugar substitute for subjects with impaired glucose tolerance or mild diabetes."[5]

The Karachi Study

A study to find out the relative glycemic tolerance of natural honey compared with simulated honey and D-glucose using oral glucose tolerance tested up to 180 minutes was carried out by researchers from several departments at the University of Karachi in Pakistan. The study was reported in *Journal of Food Science* in 2009.

Twenty-six healthy participants were randomly divided into three groups: natural honey consumers (NHC; n = 13), simulated honey consumers (AHC; n = 6), and D-glucose consumers (DGC; n = 7). After recording fasting blood glucose, the participants ate natural honey, simulated honey, or D-glucose in quantities of 1 gram per kilogram of body weight.

Subsequently, additional plasma glucose levels (PGLs) were recorded at 60, 120, and 180 minutes. At 60 minutes DGC and AHC group members exhibited similar PGL elevation (that is, 52 percent and 47 percent, respectively) compared to the NHC group with only a 20 percent increase. On the other hand, after 180 minutes, a 20 percent decrease in PGL was observed in the DGC group compared to a 9.75 percent reduction in the NHC group.

The authors concluded: "Posthoc tests showed that glucose response was significantly lower in the NHC group at all time points ($p < 0.005$) compared to the AHC and DGC groups. In conclusion, natural honey stabilizes physiological glycemic response with rebound recovery of PGL."[6]

A View from the Diet and Human Performance Laboratory—USDA

Speaking at the First International Symposium on Honey and Human Health in January 2008 in Sacramento, California, Dr. David Baer, research physiologist at the Diet and Human Performance Laboratory, USDA Agriculture Research Service, gave a presentation entitled "The Challenges of Insulin Resistance—Does Honey Have a Role?"

In addition to citing the findings of the Indian study mentioned above, Dr. Baer noted that diabetics generally have increased oxidative stress as the result of increased oxidative damage of cellular DNA, lipids, and proteins. In addition, diabetics are prone to increased vascular damage and impaired vascular function. He stated that antioxidants may be beneficial for diabetics and could help to improve endothelial function (the layer of flat cells lining the inside of blood vessels, lymphatic vessels, and the heart) and vascular (blood vessel) health. He concluded that the small amounts of antioxidants in honey may be beneficial in reducing oxidative stress. He postulated that this benefit may frequently be greater than can be explained by the actual amount of measurable antioxidants found in honey itself.[7]

Recommendations

No one is suggesting that we begin eating honey in the same amounts we eat other sugars, which is estimated at between two to three pounds (0.9–1.4 kilograms) a week. Yet the above findings would indicate that honey may be a better choice of sweetener than refined sugar or high-fructose corn syrup, especially when consumed in moderation.

Unlike the "empty" calories found in sucrose, glucose, and fructose, honey is a nutritious food. It is likely that future research will uncover more of the hidden properties of honey that contribute to its ability to help control blood-sugar levels.

12

HONEY AND
WELLNESS

*Honey's many benefits are interrelated, much like the cells
of a honeycomb, and at the very least, there are no known
medical reasons not to enjoy honey as part of a healthy
diet and lifestyle for adults and children over the age of
twelve months.*

RONALD FESSENDEN, M.D., M.P.H.

In the previous chapters I discussed how honey is a powerful antibacterial
agent that can be used to heal wounds, burns, eye infections, and internal
health problems like insomnia, gastritis, and ulcer. Yet honey can also be
of great benefit to healthy people, including athletes, people who want to
maintain their health, and for those who want to stay young despite the
number of their years. To quote the adage: "To die young, but live as long
as possible."

Much of mainstream medicine today focuses on curing disease
rather than maintaining good health. And while a growing number of
naturopaths and allopathic physicians are using honey for crisis care,
some believe that eating honey as part of one's daily routine can do
much to strengthen the body's natural immune defenses and fight off
disease. Over time, this can help us enjoy longer and healthier lives.

Much of the laboratory and clinical research presented in this book can be viewed in the light of preventive health care, although the research itself was inspired by the quest to help cure disease.

At the present time, "disease care" is placing ever-increasing pressure on health insurance companies and national health care budgets. This ultimately impacts on the health care consumer, whether directly through higher costs for medical care, or indirectly through higher insurance premiums and taxes.

Honey and Sound Nutrition

In chapter 2 I mentioned that honey is composed primarily of carbohydrates and water. It also includes small amounts of a wide variety of vitamins, including niacin, riboflavin, and pantothenic acid, along with minerals like calcium, copper, iron, magnesium, manganese, phosphorus, potassium, and zinc. In chapter 5 I also spoke about the numerous phytochemicals found in honey that are originally derived from plants. These include a wide variety of phenolics, peptides, organic acids, vitamins, and enzymes that stimulate the immune system and help kill bacteria and viruses.

Honey: A Source of Bioavailable Antioxidants

Nutritionists teach that consuming more antioxidant-rich foods may help protect our bodies from cellular damage from free radicals. Antioxidants have the unique ability to scavenge free radicals and absorb molecular damage that might otherwise compromise the function of essential nutrients like lipids and proteins, as well as nucleic acids, which carry genetic information as well as form structures within cells. Antioxidants may also help delay the aging process and prevent the development of degenerative health problems like heart disease and certain forms of cancer.

Honey contains numerous compounds with antioxidant potential. The amount and type of these antioxidant compounds depends largely upon the floral source and or variety of the honey. I mentioned earlier that darker honeys—like buckwheat and manuka—tend to be higher in antioxidants than lighter honeys, such as sage, clover, and fireweed. There is no question that the antioxidant content of honey doesn't compare with the amount found in antioxidant-rich fruits (like berries and citrus fruits) and vegetables (like broccoli, cauliflower, and kale). Yet honey provides a reliable additional source of nutritional antioxidants that are easy for the body to digest and utilize.

A major study at the Department of Nutrition at the University of California, Davis, found that honey with high levels of antioxidants may provide healthy participants protection from free radicals. The researchers took forty volunteers and divided them into four equal groups. All abstained from antioxidant-rich foods for a twenty-four-hour period before the trial, as well as throughout the experiment itself. Group one was given a basic meal of bread and water, and groups two to four were given a control meal plus corn syrup, low-antioxidant buckwheat honey, and high-antioxidant buckwheat honey, respectively.

After the meal, blood plasma levels were measured, and the researchers found that plasma total phenolic levels increased as did antioxidant and free radical–reducing capacities. The researchers concluded:

> These data support the concept that phenolic antioxidants from processed honey are bioavailable, and that they increase antioxidant activity of plasma. It can be speculated that these compounds may augment defenses against oxidative stress and they might be able to protect humans from oxidative stress. Given the average sweetener intake by humans is estimated to be in excess of 70 kg per year, the substitution of honey in some foods for traditional sweeteners could result in an enhanced antioxidant system in healthy adults.[1]

Honey and Calcium Absorption

In 2004 the Surgeon General of the United States estimated that by the year 2020, half of all Americans over the age of fifty would be at risk for osteoporosis or low bone mass. One of the most effective strategies for reducing the likelihood of osteoporosis is to consume adequate calcium.

However, one of the problems is that not all dietary calcium is easily absorbed. Some dietary factors shown to enhance the absorption of calcium include vitamin D and the sugars found in honey.

In 2005 Dr. Berdine Martin and other researchers at Purdue University showed that honey enhanced calcium absorption in laboratory animals: the more honey they consumed, the more the absorption of calcium was increased. The study, funded by the National Honey Board, was presented at the Federation of American Societies for Experimental Biology meeting in San Diego in April 2005. It showed that compared to the control group, which was given calcium and a glucose-sucrose mixture and raffinose to resemble honey, rats fed 800 mg and 500 mg of honey showed a 33.6 percent and 25.5 percent increase in calcium absorption, respectively.[2] Although these findings need to be confirmed with human subjects, they are significant because calcium deficiency is a major nutritional problem, especially among women.

Honey and Selenium Absorption

Selenium has recently gained attention for its role as an antioxidant. An important micronutrient, selenium is a component of glutathione peroxidases, a family of antioxidant enzymes that aid in preventing lipid peroxidation and membrane damage that can result from free radicals.

Studies have shown that getting enough selenium depends on the foods we eat (selenium is found primarily in nuts, cereals, meat, fish, and eggs) as well as the selenium content of the soil from which the given food originates.

A study carried out by researchers at the Medical Academy of Bialystok in Poland involving 129 individuals assessed which foods or food groups best affect serum selenium in subjects with low selenium (i.e., selenium concentrations of less than 70 micrograms per liter of blood). The researchers found that the consumption of ham, honey, and tea was positively associated with the selenium concentration in the blood of selenium-inadequate subjects.[3]

Honey, Prebiotics, and Friendly Bacteria

The gastrointestinal tract is full of bacteria that are required for proper digestion. These bacteria are essential for life and good health. One group of bacteria that has been shown to be particularly important to the health and proper function of the gastrointestinal tract is bifidobacteria. They not only aid in digestion but also are associated with increased immune levels and a lower incidence of allergies. They may also prevent the growth of certain types of cancerous tumors.

There are two basic ways to increase the populations of bifidobacteria in the gastrointestinal tract. The first method is to ingest live and active bifidobacteria cultures (such as those found in certain brands of yogurt). The other approach is to enhance the growth of the indigenous bifidobacteria itself. The first method is referred to as probiotic while the second is considered prebiotic.

Prebiotics are functional foods that increase the growth and activity of good bacteria. Most potential prebiotics are carbohydrates (such as oligosaccharides), and honey contains them in abundance. Research conducted at Michigan State University showed that adding honey to dairy products such as yogurt can enhance the growth, activity, and viability of bifidobacteria in the gastrointestinal tract.[4]

Honey and Sports Nutrition

Honey has long been recognized as one of the finest of nature's energy foods. Bernarr MacFadden, the influential founder of "Physical Culture," who combined bodybuilding with nutritional and health theories, is said to have walked the twenty-three miles from his home to his office barefoot every morning, sustained by only a glass of water with a spoonful of honey in it.

The benefits of eating carbohydrates prior to, during, and following endurance exercise are well documented. In addition, recent research supports the benefit of eating carbs prior to and during short-duration, high-intensity exercise, such as soccer, swimming competitions, and high-volume resistance training like weightlifting.

Carbohydrates eaten before and during exercise help maintain blood glucose levels and prevent premature fatigue. After exercise, carbohydrates are necessary to replenish muscle and liver glycogen and help prepare the athlete for the next training session.

Pre-Exercise

Honey may be one of the most effective ways to consume carbs before exercise. The lower glycemic index profile of honey (the glycemic index of foods refers to how quickly insulin is released by the pancreas to process the sugars they contain) is an important consideration for athletes. When honey is eaten just before exercise, it provides needed energy but also delays the release of insulin into the bloodstream and slows down the use of glycogen (muscle fuel). The end result is improved performance without the dangers of hypoglycemia.

During Exercise

Research showed that honey can improve performance during long-distance cycling trials. A study undertaken by Dr. Richard Kreider and his colleagues at the University of Memphis Exercise and Sports Nutrition Laboratory and published in the *Strength and Conditioning Journal* found that honey produced a statistically significant reduction in the trial participants' times. It also measured a significant increase in the athletes' average power when compared to a placebo. In these trials honey performed as well as glucose, the most common carbohydrate supplement used in athletics.[5]

Post-Exercise

Other studies by Dr. Kreider showed that honey is an optimal source of carbs in addition to post-workout protein supplements. Dr. Kreider found that when subjects were given one of several sweeteners after an intensive weight-training workout, those who received honey did not display the drop in blood-sugar levels after sixty minutes that affected other participants.

In addition to promoting muscle recuperation and glycogen restoration, honey-protein combinations sustain favorable blood-sugar concentrations after training that help promote recovery. Commenting on his early research, Dr. Kreider said:

> Our data suggest that honey functions well in all of the aspects associated with post-workout recuperation and energy repletion. In addition, honey appears to stand out as perhaps a better source

of carbohydrate to ingest with post-workout protein supplements. These findings support our previous study presented at the annual Experimental Biology meeting in April 2000.[6]

His early findings were borne out in more recent research in his current post as director of the Exercise and Sport Nutrition Laboratory and Center for Exercise, Nutrition, and Preventive Health Research at Baylor University. In an article he and his colleagues wrote for the November 2007 issue of the *Journal of the International Society of Sports Nutrition* about ingesting protein with various forms of carbohydrate following resistance-exercise, they reported that honey maintained blood glucose levels to a better degree than sucrose or maltodextrin.[7]

Honey and Exercise: A Few Suggestions
Remember that it is important to stay hydrated during and after exercise. In place of glucose sports drinks, add a squeeze of honey to your water bottle. You can also bring packets of honey, honey drops, or honey sticks with you when you go for a long walk or run.

If you're an athlete in training, one tablespoon of honey in warm water, lemon juice, or tea before athletic activity is considered enough to increase your energy level. For soccer, basketball, volleyball, and hockey players: take one tablespoon one-half hour before the match. You can also take one teaspoon of honey in a glass of lemon juice during rest periods. For swimmers, take one tablespoon of honey one-half hour before competition. Runners can eat a tablespoon of honey twenty minutes before the event. Cyclists can take a teaspoon of honey at mealtimes and in the form of honey sticks at regular intervals during cycling.

Honey: Key to a Restful Night's Sleep?
In the United States alone, more than 40 million are chronically ill with various sleep disorders and an additional 20 to 30 million experience intermittent sleep-related problems.

The U.S. National Commission on Sleep Disorders reports that the consequences of sleep disorders are diverse, serious, and can even be catastrophic. While there are no well-established databases on the cost of sleep disorders and sleep deprivation, the Commission was able to definitely assign 15.9 billion dollars as direct cost of sleep disorders and sleep deprivation each year. They also estimated that there were 50 to 100 billion dollars in indirect and related costs when the cost of individual accidents associated with sleep disorders and sleep deprivation are assessed including litigation, destruction of property, hospitalization, and death were taken into account. Lack of quality sleep has been linked to a wide variety of health problems, including obesity, diabetes, hypertension, memory problems and other cognitive dysfunction, depression, and other neuro-degenerative disorders.

At the present time millions of Americans are taking both prescribed and over-the-counter medications to promote sleep. In addition to the high expense, there are dangers of dependency and adverse drug reactions, especially if these drugs interact with other medications. The untimely death of actor Heath Ledger in January 2008 was determined to have been due to an accidental overdose of prescribed painkillers, sleeping pills, anti-anxiety medication, and other prescription drugs.[8]

Honey and Sleep

Honey has been used as a popular sleep aid for thousands of years. An ancient Chinese saying calls for "eating honey every night," and European folk healers have recommended drinking a cup of warm milk with honey before bedtime since the Middle Ages.

Another old-fashioned remedy is to take two teaspoons of cider vinegar with two teaspoons of honey in a glass of warm water before bedtime, while traditional Mexican healers have long prescribed a teaspoon of raw honey in a cup of warm *té de manzanilla,* or chamomile tea. Variations include a teaspoon of honey in a cup of hot water, a teaspoon of honey in a cup of passionflower tea, or simply a smear of honey on a peanut-butter sandwich before bedtime.

Honey, Sleep, and the HYMN Cycle

Scottish pharmacist, researcher, and author Mike McInnes believes that honey improves, facilitates, and lengthens restorative sleep by at least three mechanisms. When taken before bedtime, he teaches that honey:

- Ensures adequate liver-glycogen stores for eight hours of sleep. This prevents or limits the early-morning release of two stress hormones, cortisol and adrenaline.
- Stabilizes blood-sugar levels.
- Contributes to the release of melatonin, the hormone required for both the recovery and rebuilding of body tissues during rest.

The mechanism for this process can be explained by what McInnes calls the Honey-Insulin-Melatonin Cycle, or "HYMN Cycle." The cycle is described in detail in his revolutionary book *The Hibernation Diet,* co-authored with his son Stuart (see the resources).

How does the HYMN Cycle work? In a lecture and poster presentation at the First International Symposium on Honey and Human Health on January 8, 2008, McInnes described this complex process, which begins with the ingestion of one to two tablespoons of honey in the hour prior to bedtime.

The glucose portion of honey is digested and passes into the general blood circulation, producing a mild glucose spike. This mild elevation in blood sugar causes the pancreas to release a small amount of insulin into the bloodstream. This in turn drives tryptophan (an essential amino acid) into the brain, where it is converted to serotonin, a key hormone that promotes relaxation.

McInnes teaches that in darkness, serotonin is converted to melatonin in the pineal gland. (The melatonin signal forms part of the system that regulates the sleep-wake cycle by chemically causing drowsiness and lowering the body's temperature.) McInnes also stresses that melatonin inhibits the release of insulin from the pancreas, thus preventing a rapid drop in blood-sugar level.

He points out that melatonin also promotes the release of growth hormone "by another of the curious and roundabout routes that the human system excels in. The release of growth hormone is controlled by the activity of a growth-hormone-releasing hormone. This hormone is in turn inhibited by another hormone—growth-hormone-releasing-hormone-inhibiting hormone. Melatonin inhibits this last hormone, thus preventing the inhibition of growth-hormone-releasing hormone, and therefore promoting the release of growth hormone from the pituitary gland. Growth hormone is the hormone governing all of recovery physiology. This is the key first step in recovery or restorative physiology that occurs overnight."[9]

Liver glycogen, the molecule that functions as the secondary long-term energy storage in animal cells, also plays a role. The liver takes up fructose from honey, where some is converted to glucose and then to liver glycogen, thus providing the brain with a sustained supply of glucose for the night fast. McInnes maintains that the production of adequate glycogen by the liver can eliminate the release of stress hormones normally released by the adrenal glands to maintain fuel supply to the brain.

He prescribes taking one to two tablespoons of honey an hour before bedtime in order to activate the HYMN Cycle: "With the consumption of honey before bedtime, sleep quality is improved, recovery (fat burning) physiology is optimized, and the chronic release of adrenal stress hormones is inhibited."[10]

The possibility that honey can be used as a safe, inexpensive, and effective sleep aid is exciting. Further research is needed in this important field with carefully controlled and randomized human trials. A selection of honey recipes to help induce a restful night's sleep can be found in chapter 14.

13

THE FUTURE OF HONEY RESEARCH

Eating for your health has never been sweeter.
KEVIN HUGHES AND MELISSA MCALLISTER

Since the late 1990s I have witnessed a tremendous interest in the medicinal value of honey. The exponential increase in infections by antibiotic-resistant pathogens like MRSA and others have forced the medical and scientific community to take a new look at honey's numerous properties as a safe, effective, inexpensive, and easily obtainable healing agent. At the same time, a number of companies have developed creams, ointments, and bandages that incorporate healing honey. While all of them are not yet available in pharmacies throughout the world, many can be obtained through the Internet.

It is very likely that research on the therapeutic value of honey will continue to grow during the next decade. What will constitute the next frontier in honey research?

The First International Symposium on Honey and Human Health

On January 8, 2008, nearly 200 individuals—including beekeepers, honey enthusiasts, physicians, writers, and scholars from around the world—

met at a hotel in Sacramento, California, to attend the First International Symposium on Honey and Human Health. Scientists and researchers from Sweden, New Zealand, Australia, the United Kingdom, Switzerland, Israel, and the United States presented research and original work in the areas of history, health, and the microbiology of honey, as well as why it helps heal so many health problems and the numerous clinical applications for honey.

In the final presentation of the one-day symposium, Dr. Ronald Fessenden, cochairman of the Committee for the Promotion of Honey and Human Health (the organizer and sponsor of the symposium), summarized future directions for honey research. The most promising categories of honey research seemed to be in the areas of:

- Restorative sleep and beneficial body processes during sleep ("offline processing")
- Memory and cognitive function
- Insulin resistance and blood-sugar control
- Immune system enhancement
- Antimicrobial effects

Dr. Fessenden pointed out several specific types of continued research needed to confirm many of the positive healthful benefits that were suggested or indicated by the research presented in the symposium. They include:

- Human observational studies (short term)
- Studies investigating the mechanisms of action of honey within the human body
- Clinical trials involving larger study groups
- Population or epidemiological studies

However, he characterized this group as expensive, fraught with many confounding variables, challenges with control cohorts, and accidental correlations. Instead, he suggested several examples of human studies that could be conducted now at minimal expense. These included:

- Sleep lab studies observing REM sleep and/or measuring cognitive abilities post-honey dosing vs. no pre-bedtime or other food ingestion

- Expansion of oral honey "tolerance" tests measuring effects on blood glucose, HA1c, triglycerides, HDL cholesterol, and insulin response compared to glucose, HFCS, and artificial sweeteners
- Additional clinical trials using honey in pre-diabetic and diabetic patients
- Studies focused on the mechanisms of action for honey in immune system enhancement

From these latter types of study results, Dr. Fessenden believed that the scientific and medical community should be able to deduce longer-term consequences of consuming honey pending the need for population or epidemiological studies. He estimated that the potential public health benefit on metabolic diseases such as obesity, childhood obesity, insulin resistance, type-II diabetes, cardiovascular disease, and neurodegenerative diseases could be enormous. Finally, he estimated that two years of focused research could have a significant impact on the health of the next generation.[1]

The Predictions of Dr. Noori S. Al-Waili, M.D.

Dr. Noori Al-Waili is a physician and research scientist based in New York City and Dubai who has published more than 160 scientific papers, many dealing with the medicinal properties of honey. He was also a speaker at the First International Conference on Medicinal Uses of Honey that took place in Malaysia in August 2006.

In an interview with *Apitherapy News* in 2006, Dr. Al-Waili offered his predictions for future honey research.

I believe that bee products will be an important part of our modern medicine and researchers will discover unidentified ingredients and their potential usefulness in various aspects of medicine. . . .

Intravenous honey will become part of future intravenous therapy and honey inhalers will be useful for respiratory diseases. Honey and bee products will be the main component of dermatological and cosmetic preparations.[2]

Waikato Honey Research Unit

The Waikato Honey Research Unit continues to engage in groundbreaking research focusing on the healing powers of honey. By the end of 2009 researchers were involved in an impressive range of ambitious projects benefiting human health as outlined below.

- Developing a method of identifying the floral sources of honey by means of their chemical composition
- Comparison of methods of identifying the floral sources of honey for their reliability
- Investigating the flavonoids in New Zealand honeys
- Identification of the oligosaccharide constituents of honey
- Finding honeys with oligosaccharide constituents that could be growth factors for probiotic bifidobacteria
- Investigating how the antimicrobial properties of honey work against bacteria, fungi, and protozoa
- Screening a wide range of floral types of honey to find any with outstanding antibacterial or antifungal properties
- Finding the best methods for assaying the antibacterial activity of honey
- Isolating and characterizing the unique antibacterial component of manuka honey
- Assessment of the effectiveness of the antibacterial properties of honey against wound-infecting species of bacteria that are a problem to treat with antibiotics
- Assessment of the effectiveness of the antimicrobial properties of honey against fungal species causing wound infections
- Clinical trials of honey as a wound dressing for leg ulcers, pressure sores, malignant wounds, skin grafts, and donor sites for skin grafts
- Developing wound dressings that will hold honey in place on wounds effectively
- Identifying the components responsible for the anti-inflammatory activity of honey

- Comparing honeys for their content of components with antioxidant activity
- Studying honey's production of hydrogen peroxide
- Investigating the action of honey in stimulating the growth of tissues in wound healing
- Clinical trial of honey in ophthalmology
- Clinical trial of honey for treating eczema
- Trials of honey to treat acne
- Assessment of the effectiveness of the antimicrobial properties of honey against disease-causing protozoal species such as *Giardia, Cryptosporidium,* and *Trichomonas*
- Assessment of the effectiveness of the antibacterial properties of honey against bacterial species involved in gingivitis and halitosis[3]

The healing powers of honey have become far better known than ever before, and scientific and clinical research have moved forward in a wide area of study and the development of therapeutic applications. By 2010 honey was slowly gaining wider acceptance by mainstream physicians as a scientifically based, clinically measurable health care modality. Several major developments have helped create this new and exciting paradigm.

The development of honey-based medicines like Medihoney and Apinate dressings—and their approval by regulatory agencies in Europe and the United States—has far-reaching clinical possibilities. As a result, a growing number of health care providers have begun utilizing these products to treat wounds, infections, and burns in medical clinics and hospitals alike. In the United States, some of the most prestigious medical centers in the country were using honey in clinical practice, including the Mayo Clinic, the Cleveland Clinic, and teaching hospitals at Temple University, Georgetown University, and UCLA (University of California, Los Angeles).[4] Hopefully, their success will encourage other universities and medical centers in the United States and abroad to develop research programs of their own.

There are promising developments for the future. Of special note is the "honey nebulizer" for both the prevention and inhalation treatment of tuberculosis, Valley Fever, and other antibiotic-resistant pulmonary infections. Although this device received several patents in 2008, clinical trials to establish efficacy and treatment protocols are needed to determine its safety and effectiveness.

As we have seen throughout this book, honey has a wide range of healing applications. The potential public health benefit on metabolic diseases such as obesity, childhood obesity, insulin resistance, type-2 diabetes, cardiovascular disease, and neuro-degenerative diseases could be enormous, and research into the clinical applications of honey to fight these diseases provides great promise.

The continued development of "over the counter" ointments, creams, and salves by Comvita, The Honey Collection, and other companies will increase the range of honey-based elixirs, first-aid creams, burn ointments, dental hygiene products, and beauty creams that will provide consumers with natural products that are safe and effective to promote personal wellness and improved health.

Future Acceptance?

In addition to their adverse side effects, many modern drugs (especially antibiotics) have not only become ineffective against drug-resistant bacteria, but they are also helping to create new strains of "superbugs" that don't respond to traditional medicines.

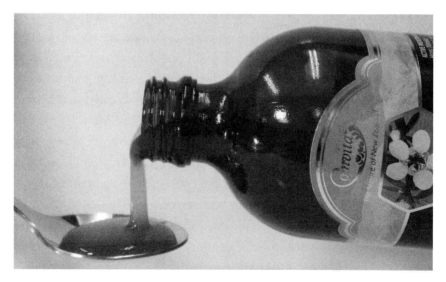

Figure 13.1. Comvita Elixir. Photo courtesy of the Comvita Medical Group.

As we've seen in earlier chapters, honey has been scientifically and clinically proven to fight these superbugs, and future clinical research will confirm and expand its range of clinical applications. I mentioned before that the main reason why these therapies have not been used to their full potential is that there is little financial incentive for physicians and pharmaceutical companies. Yet as governments continue to focus on cutting health care costs the economy, safety, and clinical effectiveness of medical-grade honey will make its use more accepted by both the medical community and the health care consumer. Long ignored and misunderstood, honey is beginning to be viewed in a new and more promising light by both patients and physicians. Hopefully this will lead to more serious study and eventual recognition by mainstream physicians and government health agencies around the world.

PART III

Honey Remedies and Recipies

A Selected Compendium for Health, Wellness, and Beauty

14

HONEY REMEDIES

There are literally thousands of folk and natural remedies that address a wide range of health problems. Many of these remedies consist of honey alone or include honey in combination with other healing elements like cinnamon and chamomile.

I am including a selection of honey remedies in this chapter as an informational guide. The remedies, approaches, and techniques described here are meant to supplement, and not to be a substitute for, professional medical care or treatment. They should not be used to treat a serious injury or health problem without prior consultation with a qualified health care professional.

External Applications

▓ Abrasions and Irritations

Treatment 1

Combine three tablespoons of honey and three tablespoons of apple-cider vinegar. Pat on the affected part with cotton. Repeat every four hours until problem resolves.

Treatment 2

Mix one teaspoon of petroleum jelly or cod liver oil with four teaspoons of honey. Mix. Apply to cuts and skin abrasions.

▩ Arthritis

Add one tablespoon of honey to two tablespoons of lukewarm water. Then add a small amount of cinnamon powder and stir into a paste. Massage the paste into the painful area.

▩ Bee Sting

Apply honey directly to the sting area.

▩ Minor Burns

Treatment 1

Immediately cool the burn with cold water. Place one tablespoon of raw honey on a sterile gauze pad and apply to burn. Change dressing several times a day.

Treatment 2

Combine one tablespoon of honey with one tablespoon of baking soda. Spread mixture over burn and cover with a sterile gauze pad.

Treatment 3

Combine two tablespoons of honey with one tablespoon of water and two tablespoons of cornstarch. Mix into a smooth paste. Apply to burn and cover with a sterile gauze pad.

▩ Bruises

Mix an equal amount of raw honey and olive oil. Apply to bruise and cover with a gauze bandage. Change dressing every four hours.

▩ Fever Blisters

When you feel that a fever blister is about to appear, apply a small amount of raw honey to the area several times a day and before going to sleep at night.

▩ Pink Eye

Place two tablespoons of warm water in a glass and add one tablespoon of honey. Take some toilet paper or tissue and fashion into a one-inch by three-inch strip. Dip the corner of the paper into the mixture and squeeze a few drops into the infected eye. There may be a slight burning sensation. Close your eye for two minutes. Treatment can be done several times a day for two or three days.

Sunburn and Chafing Ointment

Combine two tablespoons of honey, two tablespoons of glycerin, two tablespoons of lemon juice, and one tablespoon of rubbing alcohol in a jar. Shake well until mixed. Apply to affected area as needed.

Honey Paste for Wounds

Take ten parts (by weight) of beeswax and add three parts of propolis extract (10 percent ethanol) and two parts of raw honey. Melt the wax and, while it is cooling, add the propolis and the honey. Mix well. Then place the mixture in a jar and store in a cool dry place. You can apply the paste to treat many types of skin wounds, infections, burns, and sores; you can also chew the paste to help relieve mouth and gum infections.

Internal Applications

Remember that honey's inhibine factor is reduced if it is heated to more than 104°F (40°C). For this reason, healers recommend either keeping the temperature of the liquid to which honey is added under this level or using manuka honey—which does not lose its antimicrobial powers when heated—instead.

Arthritis

Treatment 1

Take one cup of hot water with two teaspoons of honey and one level teaspoon of ground cinnamon in the morning and again at night.

Treatment 2

Combine one tablespoon of honey with one-half teaspoon of ground cinnamon. Take before breakfast.

▓ Asthma

Take one stick of cinnamon, two tablespoons of thyme, one lime (halved), three heads of garlic (peeled), and one-half a purple onion (chopped), and place the ingredients into two cups of water and bring to a boil. Then add another cup of water. Continue to boil until the mixture reduces to half. Strain. Add one teaspoon of honey and drink one cup as a tea three times a day. You can also add honey to taste and serve the tea as a medicine: take one tablespoon every three hours, with the last dose as close to bedtime as possible.

▓ Bladder Infections

Add two tablespoons of ground cinnamon and one teaspoon of honey to a glass of lukewarm water. Drink two to three times a day.

▓ High Blood Pressure

Take one teaspoon of garlic juice mixed with two teaspoons of honey. Take twice a day: once in the morning and again in the evening. Take on a regular basis.

▓ Blood Purification and Fat Reduction

To help purify the blood and clean the bowels, take a glass of warm water and add one to two teaspoonfuls of honey with one teaspoonful of lemon juice. Take this preparation daily before going to the bathroom.

▓ Colitis

Dissolve three tablespoons of honey in a glass of lukewarm water. Drink in the evening.

▓ Colds

Treatment 1

Combine one tablespoon of warm honey with one-quarter teaspoon of ground cinnamon. Take once or twice daily for three days.

Treatment 2

Add one teaspoon of honey to a cup of herbal tea or warm milk. Drink three to four cups a day.

Treatment 3

Add one teaspoon of honey to an eight-ounce cup of warm water and take three times a day.

Treatment 4

Take one one-quarter-inch slice of onion and mince, two cloves of crushed garlic, two tablespoons of honey, and one-quarter teaspoon of crushed dry red pepper and mix together. Take one or two teaspoons before meals for two to three days.

Treatment 5

This Mexican cold remedy calls for boiling five cloves of freshly minced garlic in two cups of water. Allow to cool until warm. Add one teaspoon of honey and a slice of lemon or lime. Drink two times daily for three days.

Treatment 6

Take two cups of hot water and add two teaspoons of chamomile leaves. Allow to cool. Add one tablespoon of honey and three teaspoons of lemon juice. Drink two times daily for three days.

Treatment 7

This novel New Zealand remedy involves honey, lemon juice, and whiskey. Squeeze the juice from one lemon into a cup and add one tablespoon of manuka honey. Add a tablespoon of whiskey and mix together. Fill the glass with hot water and allow to cool. Drink one cup daily for three days.

▨ Constipation

Treatment 1

Prepare a bowl of freshly cut fruit and add one tablespoon of honey. Consume at least three times daily.

Treatment 2

Upon rising in the morning, add one tablespoon of honey to a twelve-ounce glass of lukewarm water. Drink on an empty stomach.

▦ Cough

Treatment I

Mix one teaspoon of honey and one teaspoon of ginger juice. Take two to three times a day as needed. It immediately relieves symptoms of cold, cough, sore throat, chest congestion, and runny nose.

Treatment 2

For cough or fever, add a quarter teaspoon of fresh lime or lemon juice and mix with one teaspoon of honey added to an eight-ounce cup of warm water. Take four times a day.

Treatment 3

This traditional ayurvedic remedy is recommended especially for dry cough. Mix one tablespoon of honey with one-third teaspoon of powdered turmeric. Lick mixture off the spoon.

Treatment 4

Add a tablespoon of fresh lemon juice to one-quarter cup of raw honey. Take a teaspoon of the mixture every two or three hours.

Treatment 5

This unusual cough remedy calls for one large onion. Slice it in half. Remove the inner eight or nine layers of the onion (to use later for cooking or a salad) and pour raw honey into the cavity. Place the onion and honey into a refrigerator for three hours. Remove. Take three teaspoons of honey every two hours until cough subsides.

A variation calls for one medium-size chopped onion. Pour one tablespoon of honey over the onion and allow to stand for four hours. Take one teaspoon of the juice every hour, or as needed to relieve coughing.

Treatment 6, Bronchitis and Whooping Cough

To relieve cough and wheezing associated with bronchitis or whooping cough, mix one teaspoon of finely chopped thyme with one tablespoon of honey. Take as needed.

Treatment 7

Dr. Maoshing Ni, author of *Secrets of Self-Healing* (Avery, 2007), suggests that to soothe a cough, core and peel one Asian pear (easily available in food markets that specialize in Asian products). Add one tablespoon of honey to the center. Steam or bake for ten to fifteen minutes. Eat two to three times a day.

▓ Depression

Treatment 1
Drink a cup of warm milk sweetened with honey before bedtime.

Treatment 2
Prepare a mug of chamomile tea and add one teaspoon of honey and one-half teaspoon of bee pollen. Drink before bedtime.

▓ Diarrhea

Treatment 1
To treat diarrhea, add one teaspoon of honey to eight ounces of barley water. Take three times a day.

Treatment 2
Dissolve four tablespoons of honey in one pint of lukewarm water. Drink one-half cup as needed. Not recommended for diabetics.

▓ Digestive Problems (Upset Stomach, Gastritis)

Treatment 1
Add one teaspoon of honey to one cup of warm chamomile or linden flower tea. Drink three times daily.

Treatment 2
Add one teaspoon of honey to one cup of naturally carbonated mineral water. Add lemon or lime if desired. Take as needed.

Treatment 3
Take one tablespoon of honey upon rising in the morning and another before going to bed at night.

Treatment 4
Take three tablespoons of honey daily, either alone or mixed with other foods. It can also be combined with lukewarm water. Mexican folk heal-

ers suggest consuming honey as medicine two hours before breakfast and three hours after dinner.

Treatment 5

To facilitate healing of gastritis and stomach ulcers, take one to two teaspoons of UMF-10+ Manuka honey three to four times per day, fifteen to twenty minutes before meals.

Treatment 6

Combine twenty-five fresh mint leaves (or one teaspoon dried) with twenty-five fresh rosemary leaves (or one teaspoon dried). Add to a quart of hot water and allow to cool. After one hour, add three tablespoons of honey and mix. Allow to steep for twenty-four hours. Strain. Take one-half cup before bed, either cold or warm.

Treatment 7

Sprinkle ground cinnamon on two tablespoons of honey and take before meals. This will aid in the digestion of even the heaviest of foods.

Elevated Cholesterol

Take sixteen ounces (.47 liters) of warm water and add two tablespoons of honey and three teaspoons of ground cinnamon. Mix together and drink as a tea three times a day.

Hay Fever

When we eat local honey, we are ingesting pollen from local plants. Over time this may have a desensitizing effect and may help reduce our allergic reaction to pollen when we breathe it in. Take at least one teaspoon of locally harvested honey a day either right from the jar or in tea, over cereal, or on toast. It's best to begin taking this remedy one month before allergy season begins.

Heart Tonic

Treatment I

Combine one teaspoon of anise powder with one or two teaspoons of honey. It is believed to strengthen the heart and improve its functioning.

Treatment 2

Another heart remedy calls for substituting honey mixed with ground cinnamon to be used instead of jelly or jam on bread.

Treatment 3

Take one teaspoon of honey and add to one cup of warm water. Mix and take two or three times a day.

▦ Herpes

Add three teaspoons of honey to one teaspoon of cod liver oil. Mix thoroughly and apply to the affected area as often as needed.

▦ Insomnia

Treatment 1

Add one teaspoon of honey to one cup of warm chamomile, orange blossom, lemon balm, or linden flower tea. Drink before bedtime.

Treatment 2

Add one teaspoon of honey to one cup of warm milk. Drink before bedtime.

Treatment 3

Prepare half a glass of orange juice diluted with an equal amount of lukewarm water. Add two teaspoons of honey and drink just before bedtime.

Treatment 4

Add one teaspoon of honey to a cup of warm peppermint tea. A clove can be added if desired.

Treatment 5

Combine two ounces (55 grams) of honey with five drops of lavender oil. Add one or two tablespoons of this mixture to a warm tub of water and enjoy a relaxing soak for ten to fifteen minutes.

▦ Kidney Problems

Make a fresh juice with two large radishes and add one tablespoon of honey. Repeat dosage at least once.

▦ *Laryngitis*

Drink large amounts of warm milk or tea sweetened with honey. Or simply take three teaspoons of honey a day.

▦ *Liver Problems*

Mix two tablespoons of honey into a bowl containing cottage cheese, cooked cereal, and small pieces of fresh apple. Eat twice a day.

▦ *To Promote Longevity*

One ayurvedic remedy calls for adding one tablespoon of honey and one-quarter teaspoon of ground cinnamon to one-half cup of hot water. Drink three to four times daily.

▦ *Sore Throat*

Treatment 1

Squeeze one whole lemon into a cup. Add a teaspoon of honey, a pinch of salt, and two tablespoons of apple cider vinegar. Mix together and swallow.

Treatment 2

Brew a cup of orange pekoe tea. Add one tablespoon of honey and two tablespoons of lemon juice. Drink three times a day. A similar remedy suggests brewing a cup of chamomile tea and adding the juice of one lemon and three to four teaspoons of honey.

Treatment 3

Combine one teaspoon of apple cider vinegar, one teaspoon of cayenne pepper, and three tablespoons of raw honey. Add to a cup of warm water. Use as a gargle as often as necessary.

Treatment 4

Brew a cup of warm sage tea and add one teaspoon of honey and one teaspoon of apple cider vinegar. Use as a gargle.

Treatment 5

Combine two tablespoons of buckwheat honey, two tablespoons of glycerin, two tablespoons of lemon juice, and one-eighth teaspoon of ground ginger. Place in a bowl or Pyrex jar and warm in hot water. Place in a bottle, cork, and shake well. Sip at regular intervals to soothe a sore throat.

Treatment 6

Add a tablespoon of fresh lemon juice to one-quarter cup of raw honey. Take a teaspoon of the mixture every two or three hours for sore throat.

Tonsillitis

Mix five drops of fresh lemon juice into one tablespoon of honey. Take every three hours until symptoms disappear.

Toothache

Take one teaspoon of ground cinnamon and five teaspoons of honey and mix into a paste. Spread on a piece of bread and apply on the aching tooth. This may be done three times a day or until pain subsides.

15

HONEY:
KEY TO BEAUTY

Other bees, like soldiers, armed in their stings,
Make boot upon the summer's velvet buds,
Which pillage they with merry march bring home.
WILLIAM SHAKESPEARE, *KING HENRY V*

Humans have used honey to help maintain healthy skin and hair for thousands of years. Legend has it that Cleopatra, the Queen of Egypt, applied honey to her face as a masque every morning and took milk and honey baths to keep her skin smooth, healthy, and young. Poppea, wife of the Roman emperor Nero, used a honey and milk lotion on her face to keep it looking youthful.

Other female historical figures knew of the beautifying properties of honey as well: women of the French royal court, including Madame du Barry, the last mistress of King Louis XV of France, were said to use honey regularly as a facial masque. In England, Queen Anne was believed to have used a secret honey and oil recipe to keep her hair thick and shiny, while Sarah, the Duchess of Marlborough, was reputed to have her own secret recipe for a special honey water she applied to her hair to keep it beautiful. In Ming dynasty China, women in the emperor's court used a blend of honey and ground orange seeds to keep their skin fresh and blemish-free.

177

The ancients prized honey as a beauty tonic because it never needed additives of any kind to keep it from spoiling. Only much later did modern scientists discover that honey has strong antioxidant properties and is a storehouse of enzymes, amino acids, and vitamins and minerals that reduce inflammation and promote cellular regeneration, which helps keep skin young.

By the late 1800s honey had become a common ingredient in many cosmetics, and today literally thousands of commercial beauty products are made with honey, especially bath and shower products, face creams, and skin lotions. According to the National Honey Board, hair care is the area where the use of honey is growing the most. In addition, it reports that researchers are developing a process that uses honey to create alpha hydroxy acids, ingredients used in skin creams and moisturizers because they help exfoliate the skin. Scientists are also developing honey-based sun-care products that combine sun blockers, moisturizers, and anti-irritants.

As can be expected, many of the world's leading health and beauty spas provide specialized skin and hair treatments with honey-based preparations. But you don't have to buy a pricey cosmetic or go to an expensive spa to enjoy the beauty-enhancing benefits of honey. Many of the following time-tested honey recipes—created by and for beauty-conscious women (and men) from around the world—are both inexpensive and simple to make.

Honey Treatments for the Skin

▓ *Pimples and Blemishes*

Treatment 1

Combine three tablespoons of honey and one teaspoon of ground cinnamon to make a paste. Apply to affected skin before sleeping, and wash it off the next morning with warm water. Estimated time of cure: two weeks.

Treatment 2

Mix one-half cup of warm water with one-quarter teaspoon of salt. Take a cotton ball or gauze and apply the salted water directly to the blemish, using light pressure. Reapply over the next several minutes to soften the blemish. Now take a cotton swab and dab a small amount of honey on the softened blemish. Allow to remain on the skin for ten minutes. Rinse with warm water and pat dry.

▦ For Radiant Skin

Treatment 1

Mix a small piece of banana with one teaspoon of honey and one-half teaspoon of yogurt. Apply to skin and leave for ten minutes. Wash off thoroughly with lukewarm water.

Treatment 2

Take the yolk of one egg and add one tablespoon of honey. Mix thoroughly. Apply to the face and neck with a soft brush or with the fingers, being careful not to get any of the mixture into the eyes. Allow it to remain for twenty minutes and then wash with lukewarm water.

Treatment 3

Add some sugar to warm water and use it to wash the face gently. Dry. Then, apply a layer of raw honey directly to the face and allow it to remain for fifteen to twenty minutes. Rinse off with warm water. For best results, use this recipe once a week.

Treatment 4

Purée one peeled and cored apple along with one tablespoon of honey in a blender. Smooth the apple and honey mixture over the face. Leave on for fifteen minutes and then rinse with cold water.

Treatment 5

With a fork, beat together one egg white, one tablespoon of honey, and one teaspoon of glycerin. Add just enough flour to form a paste. Smooth the paste over the face and throat. Leave on for ten minutes while relaxing. Rinse off with warm water.

▦ Facial Treatments

Treatment 1

Take one-third cup of raw instant oatmeal and add enough honey to make a smooth paste. Add one tablespoon of rose water or orange flower water to thin. Mix well. Spread the mixture over a clean face, being careful to avoid getting into the eyes. Leave on for thirty minutes and relax. Rinse with lukewarm water and add an astringent to the skin if desired.

Dr. Bernard Jensen's Beautifying Honey Facial

First, apply cleansing cream to the face and neck. Wash off with warm water, which will open the pores. Then pat small amounts of honey onto the face and neck with fingertips until the skin tingles and glows. Allow the honey to remain for thirty minutes while you relax. Then rinse off with warm water and finally rinse with cold water. Recommended frequency: once a week to soften skin or before special occasions.

Skin Cleansing

Treatment 1

Take two tablespoons of cooked oatmeal and mix in two tablespoons of honey and one-half tablespoon of yogurt. Apply to the face and leave for fifteen minutes. Wash with water. For best results, do every morning.

Treatment 2

Mix two tablespoons of honey with one-quarter cup of plain yogurt. Then take one-half cup of dry oatmeal and grind it until it becomes a fine powder. Add to the honey-yogurt mixture and mix until it becomes a smooth paste. Apply to the face and neck and allow to stand for fifteen minutes. Rinse with lukewarm water and pat dry.

Treatment 3

Mix two tablespoons of honey with a beaten egg white. Apply thinly to the skin and allow to dry. Rinse off with lukewarm water. This recipe is especially recommended for oily skin.

Treatment 4

Combine one-half cup of almond meal and enough honey to form a thick paste. Scrub the face with the paste, paying special attention to oily areas. Leave on for a few minutes. Remove with lukewarm water and a soft cloth.

Treatment 5

Blend two tablespoons of finely ground raw almonds with one tablespoon of honey and one-half tablespoon of fresh lemon juice. Rub the paste gently into the skin. Rinse with warm water.

Treatment 6

With a fork, beat together one egg white, one tablespoon of honey, and one teaspoon of glycerin. Add just enough flour to form a paste. Smooth the paste over the face and throat. Leave on for ten minutes while relaxing. Rinse off with warm water.

▓ *For Skin Nutrition and Moisturizing*

Treatment 1

Take one-half cup of milk and add one peeled and mashed avocado, one cooked carrot (mashed), and three tablespoons of honey. Mix together and use as a masque on the face and neck. Leave on for fifteen minutes. Wash with lukewarm water.

Treatment 2

Take one ripe banana and mash. Add one tablespoon of milk or cream, one tablespoon of honey, and the yolk of one egg. Mix thoroughly. Apply as a masque on the face and neck. Leave on for fifteen minutes. Wash with lukewarm water.

Treatment 3

Mix one teaspoon of almond oil, one tablespoon of honey, and one-quarter teaspoon of fresh lemon juice. Rub the mixture into hands, elbows, feet, or anywhere your skin feels dry. Leave on for ten minutes. Remove with lukewarm water and a soft cloth.

Treatment 4

Take one tablespoon of sweet almond oil and two tablespoons of honey. Mix together. Carefully wash the face and then apply to the skin. Allow to remain for thirty minutes while relaxing. Remove with a soft cloth and lukewarm water.

Treatment 5

Take one-half cup of instant oatmeal and add four teaspoons of honey. Mix well, adding more honey to achieve a smooth consistency. Spread over the face and allow to stand for thirty minutes. Wash off with warm water and then rinse with cold water to tighten pores.

Treatment 6

Combine one teaspoon of honey, one egg white (small), and one tablespoon of milk. Beat with a fork until smooth. Cleanse face and neck and then spread mixture over the face. Allow to remain for thirty minutes or until dry and brittle. Wash off with warm water and then splash with cold water.

▓ Antiwrinkle Applications

Treatment 1

Take one tablespoon of honey and one tablespoon of fresh lemon juice. Mix the honey and lemon juice together and gently massage the liquid into the face and neck. Allow to remain for twenty minutes. Wash carefully with a sponge or cotton ball soaked in lukewarm water.

Treatment 2

Mix one tablespoon of honey into a glass of fresh milk. Rinse face with the mixture. Allow it to dry naturally and then rinse with lukewarm water.

Treatment 3

Add two drops of fresh lemon juice to one tablespoon of honey. Mix well. Place mixture directly on the affected area and allow to stand for ten minutes. Rinse with lukewarm water.

Treatment 4

To make a good skin cream, take one teaspoon of almond oil, two drops of perfume, two tablespoons of light honey, and one small egg. Combine in a small bowl and beat until fluffy. Spoon into a small jar and store in refrigerator. Apply to the face and leave on for twenty minutes. Rinse off with lukewarm water. You can also use this cream for chapped hands.

Treatment 5

Take one-half cup of skimmed milk and add one tablespoon of honey and one teaspoon of aloe vera gel. Combine ingredients in a jar and shake well. Apply to your face morning and evening with a cotton ball. Store mixture in the refrigerator.

Skin Lotion

To make a simple skin lotion, take one teaspoon of honey, three ounces of glycerin, one and one-half ounces of lemon juice, one ounce of rubbing alcohol, and two ounces of rose water. Place in a bottle. Seal and shake vigorously. Apply to the skin as needed.

Face Cream

For a simple face cream, combine one teaspoon of honey with one well-beaten egg white and a few drops of almond oil. Mix together until you get a smooth cream. Use as needed.

Hand Cream

To make a medium-soft hand cream, blend one teaspoon of rose water with one teaspoon of olive oil, two tablespoons of honey, and two and one-half tablespoons of almond meal. Thicken with cornstarch or arrow-root if too thin. Rub well into hands as needed.

Hand Cleanser

Blend two tablespoons of finely ground corn meal with two tablespoons of honey and one tablespoon of cornstarch or arrowroot powder. Store in a jar and use as a hand soap.

Cleopatra's Milk and Honey Bath

Mix one-half cup of warm milk with one-half cup of honey and two teaspoons of jojoba oil (optional) in a bowl. Pour the mixture into your warm bath. Soak for up to twenty minutes to allow these beneficial ingredients to infuse your skin. This recipe makes enough for one bath.

As a variation, simply add one-quarter cup of honey to a bathtub full of warm water for a luxurious—if not royal—bath.

Chapped Lips

Treatment I

Add one-half teaspoon of honey to one teaspoon of petroleum jelly. Mix together thoroughly and apply to chapped lips once in the morning and once in the evening. Allow to stand for ten minutes and then rinse with warm water.

Treatment 2

Take two tablespoons of honey and add two tablespoons of lemon juice and two tablespoons of cologne. Blend together and apply to lips when needed.

▨ Honey Treatments for the Hair

Following are two recipes that can be used on the scalp before you wash your hair.

Balsam for Dry Hair

Take one tablespoon of honey and three tablespoons of olive oil (you can prepare more if you have long hair: remember to use one part honey for every three parts olive oil) and mix ingredients in a cup or glass and allow to sit for twenty-four hours. Before using, mix again, then apply to the hair, being sure to massage thoroughly into the scalp with circular movements to stimulate blood circulation. Cover the hair with a plastic shower cap and wait for thirty minutes. Then wash with lukewarm water and rinse several times; rinse the final time with a little vinegar or lemon juice.

Honey Cap

Take one-half cup of raw honey and apply directly to wet hair. Allow it to penetrate to the scalp by gentle circular massage. Cover hair with a plastic shower cap and relax for twenty minutes. Rinse hair with lukewarm water and then shampoo as usual.

Hair Shine

This recipe can be used either by those who wish to use shampoo in addition to honey or who choose not to use shampoo at all. In addition to promoting the general health of the hair and scalp, honey cleans as well.

Add one teaspoon of honey and one-quarter teaspoon of fresh lemon juice to one quart of lukewarm water. Mix. Shampoo as usual and then pour mixture through the hair. Do not rinse; dry as normal.

PART IV

Bees and the Future

16

A THREATENED
SPECIES

*You can't say that one thing is causing bees to die because
there are several things out there attacking them.*

PROFESSOR ERIC MUSSEN,
UNIVERSITY OF CALIFORNIA, DAVIS

During the months of October, November, and December 2006, an
alarming number of honeybee colonies began to die along the East Coast
of the United States. West Coast beekeepers also began to report unprec-
edented losses. By the middle of 2007, similar reports began to appear
in Latin America, Europe, and parts of Asia. Some American beekeepers
reported that up to 80 percent of their bee colonies were lost, virtually
overnight. It is believed that out of the 2.5 million beehives in the United
States, 750,000 were lost by the winter of 2007.

This phenomenon, without a recognizable underlying cause, was first
termed Fall Dwindle Disease, but was later renamed Colony Collapse
Disorder, or simply CCD. It not only threatens the pollination industry
and production of commercial honey in the United States and Canada
but also affects bee colonies in Europe and Latin America.

CCD has become a highly significant yet poorly understood problem.
Many beekeepers are openly wondering if the industry can survive. There are

serious concerns that losses are so great that there will not be enough bees to rebuild colony numbers sufficiently to maintain economic viability in these beekeeping operations, which are responsible for approximately $15 billion worth of crops a year. Because more than 70 percent of the fruits and vegetables we eat—including carrots, cucumbers, broccoli, onions, pumpkins, squash, apples, blueberries, avocados, and almonds—are pollinated by honeybees, the impact of CCD poses a major threat to the human food supply.

Some have commented that the widespread death of honeybees is like "the canary in the coal mine" and is a signal that our environment is in deep trouble. Although scientists have not been able to pinpoint one specific cause, there are a number of major suspects. When taken together, these suspected causes create a powerful indictment on the present state of agriculture in the postindustrial world and sound the alarm for radical and forceful change that will not be easy.

A Multifaceted Syndrome

There is still much speculation about the causes of CCD. Some early reports of cell-phone towers and genetically modified crops being responsible for the syndrome have been discounted. Yet several other causes remain suspect. They include a virus, drought, a parasitic mite, stress, importation of bees from foreign countries, poor nutrition, and pesticides. When examined alone, each possible cause only appears to make up a part of the picture. Yet when taken together, they create a scenario that begins to make sense.

A Virus and a Mite

The USDA Agricultural Research Service reports that the only pathogen found in almost all samples from honeybee colonies with CCD, but not in non-CCD colonies, was the Israeli acute paralysis virus (IAPV), a dicistrovirus that can be transmitted by the varroa mite. It was found in 96.1 percent of the CCD-bee samples.[1]

Stress and the Traveling Honeybee

The report also mentioned another possible cause. In earlier times bees primarily lived in the same area throughout their lives. They may have been transported by wagon from farm to farm by farmers who wanted to take advantage of the flowering of different crops during the normal growing season.

Though there are still small-scale beekeepers whose bees remain in the local bioregion, the vast majority of beekeepers are huge commercial operations involving hundreds of thousands of beehives. Like many of the huge "factory farms" that provide meat, fruit, and vegetables to the vast majority of Americans, the model of industrial agriculture has come to beekeeping as well.

Today literally billions of bees are transported throughout the country every year on the back of flatbed trucks. For example, a few million bees might spend a few weeks in New England pollinating blueberry plants; they would later be hauled to Florida to pollinate strawberry fields. As February approaches, they would be awakened from their normal hibernation cycle and transported to California's Central Valley to join more than a million other hives (containing more than 40 billion bees) to help pollinate the annual almond crop.

Many scientists postulate that the wholesale transporting of bees throughout the continent is a source of stress for the honeybees, which can reduce their ability to fight disease. According to an article by Michael Pollan in *The New York Times Magazine,* "The lifestyle of the modern

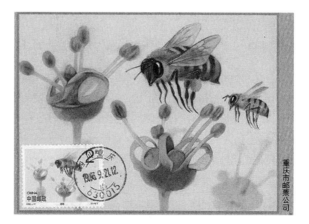

Figure 16.1. Honeybees pollinating flowers. From a postal souvenir sheet, Peoples Republic of China.

honeybee leaves the insects so stressed out and their immune system so compromised that, much like livestock on factory farms, they've become vulnerable to whatever new infectious agent happens to come along."[2] Anecdotal evidence suggests that CCD is most common among bee populations that are trucked long distances and rented out for pollination, while bees that spend their lives in the same area—and especially those who feed on organically grown plants—are the least affected.

Guest Workers from Abroad

While the press has devoted a lot of attention to undocumented agricultural workers streaming into the United States from Mexico and other parts of Latin America, the wholesale importation of worker honeybees has largely gone unnoticed. Many of these bees hail from Australia, a country where CCD has not yet become a major problem.

More than half of all the beehives in America travel to California for the almond-tree bloom every February. Because the demand for honeybees far outstrips the domestic supply, millions of "guest workers" are flown in from abroad and trucked to the Central Valley, where they mingle with the honeybees who arrive from all over North America. Referred to unceremoniously as "one big brothel" by a California beekeeper, the almond orchards are a place where bees swap microbes and parasites from all over the country and the world before they move on to new pollinating tasks in other parts of the United States and Canada. As a result, many new pathogens (and combinations of pathogens) are easily introduced to even the stay-at-home bees that don't get to labor in California's almond orchards during the winter.

The Weather

Over the past few decades global warming has produced unusual and extreme weather patterns that can affect bees and the plants they feed on, leading both scientists and beekeepers to believe that unusual weather patterns play a role in CCD.

A warmer winter than normal can send confusing signals to bees, resulting in fewer bees in flight in the spring. Drought and wildfires can prevent flowers from blooming. A late freeze in the spring can bring nectar flows in many areas almost to a halt, resulting in honeybee starvation. While there has always been a degree of variability within the natural weather patterns, we need to examine the long-term trends and the implications they may bring to the welfare of honeybees and other insects.

Poor Nutrition

I mentioned in chapter 2 that the natural foods for bees are pollen and honey. Because humans have prized both of these foods since the time of the ancient honey hunters, they are often removed from the hive and used as human foods.

Taking honey from bees has never been easy. Early honey hunters—as do modern honey harvesters—risk getting stung by angry bees that defend their hives to the death. When skeps—baskets made of coiled grass or straw—were developed to domesticate honeybees, the easiest way to gather their honey was to simply kill all of the bees and harvest whatever honey was found in the beehive.

Hive designs developed in the early 1900s made it possible for beekeepers to take only a portion of the honey and pollen from the beehive without having to kill the entire colony. Wise beekeepers usually left the bees with enough honey and pollen to survive during the winter. Many beekeepers continue to use this method today.

Yet most of the large beekeeping operations in North America today remove all the honey and pollen from the hive without killing the bees. To compensate for the honeybees' loss, they feed the bees high-fructose corn syrup and other sugar-based supplements. Many of these supplements are laced with antibiotics. Unlike honey, which contains a vast array of minute amounts of vitamins, minerals, and enzymes the bee needs for proper nourishment, these sugary mixtures are devoid of nutrients and are essentially junk food for bees.

Even when bees are able to enjoy their own honey and pollen, other problems can occur. An editorial in the *New York Times* about CCD mentioned that a period of drought, which caused the plants to produce less nectar and pollen than usual, could be a contributing factor to CCD.

As we saw in an earlier chapter, both honey and pollen are essential for good honeybee nutrition.[3]

Another nutrition-related issue has to do with the growing tendency to move bees to regions where only one type of plant is available. While the nectar and pollen from a monoculture may be perfectly good in itself, bees would naturally visit a variety of plants that provide a variety of nutrients. Even in areas where many plant species thrive, the amount of this valuable—and varied—pasture is shrinking. As a result, the honeybees do not get all the trace elements they need for good health.

According to Gloria Degrandi-Hoffman, director of the U.S. Department of Agriculture's Carl Hayden Bee Research Center in Tucson, Arizona, poor nutrition is one of the basic components of CCD. During a 2008 interview with a reporter from the *Tucson Citizen,* Dr. Hoffman said: "Something like poor nutrition will set up many things. Just like humans, if bees are not eating well they are likely to come down with illnesses and be less resistant to diseases and stresses."[4]

To help remedy this situation, scientists at the Carl Hayden Bee Research Center, as well as several enterprising beekeepers, have developed food supplements that contain a variety of nutrients, including protein, vitamins, and minerals. One California beekeeper I spoke with who developed such a supplement found that it was well tolerated by his bees and actually helped decrease the impact of CCD in his hives.

Diseases

Disease among *Apis mellifera* has been common since the honeybee was first introduced to the United States in the seventeenth century. Diseases related to parasites, bacteria, fungal infections, viral infection, dysentery, chilled brood, and pesticides have killed many thousands of bee colonies over the years. The June 18, 1884, issue of *The Weekly Bee Journal* contained a long article about curing foulbrood, a widespread and highly destructive disease caused by the spore-forming *Paenibacillus larvae* spp. The author reported that to cure foulbrood, "The foulbroody colonies [should] receive every other evening one-sixth of a litre of syrup containing 30 to 50 drops of Hilbert's solution No. 1 (8 grammes or cubic centimetres of pure alcohol to 1 gramme of salicylic acid)."[5]

Since the 1980s honeybee colony health has been declining in North America, partly due to the arrival of new pathogens and pests from other parts of the world. The spread into the United States of varroa mites and tracheal mites in particular has created major new stresses on honeybees. In addition to spreading diseases to honeybee colonies, the varroa mite sucks blood from both adult bees and the developing brood. They are big enough to be seen with the naked eye. The tracheal mite, an exotic species that arrived in America in 1987, invades the respiratory tract of bees, choking them to death.

Pesticides

As in other areas of industrial agriculture, commercial beekeepers find it necessary to treat their bees with a cocktail of medications and in-house pesticides to keep their bees healthy. Some of the pesticides are given to treat a variety of viruses and parasites like the varroa mite or the cleptoparasitic hive beetle.

In addition, bees have to contend with a wide variety of pesticides that are sprayed on nearby plants. Scientists have found that where insecticides are used, bee colony losses are common. By contrast, many beekeepers who do not use in-house chemicals or whose bees tend to feed from organically grown plants have not experienced CCD in their hives.

The death of millions of bee colonies in many parts of the world is an extremely serious problem that calls for solutions from scientists, farmers, homeowners, and beekeepers. Improving nutrition, reducing stress, and eliminating dangerous pesticides are essential first steps in creating healthier bee populations. In the following chapter we will explore these measures as well as other ways to help restore bee and other pollinator populations and create a better environment that will allow them to multiply and thrive.

17

RESTORE THE ENVIRONMENT, PROTECT THE BEES

If the bee disappears from the surface of the Earth, man would have no more than four years to live. No more bees, no more pollination . . . no more men!

ALBERT EINSTEIN

Honeybees, native bees, and other pollinating insects are a vital part of our environment and play a crucial role in the production of many of the crops we use as food. At the same time, they are important "indicators" that help us monitor the extent of environmental contamination taking place across the globe. Honeybees are extremely sensitive to pesticides, which usually results in a high bee mortality rate. In addition, residues of pesticides and other environmental contaminants (such as heavy metals and radionuclides) can be detected in their bodies or in beehive products like honey and pollen.[1]

As we saw in the previous chapter, the dramatic loss of honeybee populations in many parts of North America and other regions of the world is a systemic problem that is inseparable from industrial agriculture, a form of modern farming that involves the industrialized production of livestock, poultry, fish, and crops. This system dominates in North America and other regions of the developed world today. While it may result in cheaper food and enormous profits for agribusiness, many family farmers go out of business. And because factory farms require ever-increasing amounts of pesticides to ensure profitable yields, pollution from corporate farms degrades the environment. That is one reason why a U.S. Office of Technology Assessment conducted by the UC Davis Macrosocial Accounting Project concluded that industrial agriculture is associated with substantial deterioration of human living conditions in nearby rural communities.[2]

Changing this system is not a simple matter. According to Rowan Jacobsen, author of *Fruitless Fall: The Collapse of Honeybees and the Coming Agricultural Crisis,* "The answer is to stop using chemicals on our crops and in our hives, stop flying bees in from Australia, stop breeding bees for honey production and brood production at the expense of fitness, and to revert to a smaller, organic model of farming."[3]

The primary purpose of this book has been to focus on the therapeutic value of honey and its myriad applications in human health. Yet the overwhelming threat to both honeybees and native bee populations is intricately tied to the *protection of* honeybees and other pollinators that are vital to a healthy environment.

Protecting Honeybees from Pesticides

Protecting honeybees and other pollinators from pesticide poisoning is extremely important. While there is a definite trend away from pesticides to more natural methods of pest control, the following recommendations can help minimize bee kills. They are based on the research of Dr. James E. Tew of the Department of Entomology's Honey Bee Laboratory at Ohio State University. His complete paper on the subject can be found at the Honey Bee Lab's website (www.beelab.osu.edu/factsheets/sheets/2161 .html).

Pesticides on Blossoms

Because bees focus on the blossom of the plant, farmers should avoid spraying during the blossom period. Spraying nonblooming crops with a hazardous pesticide when nearby cover crops, weeds, or wildflowers are in bloom may also be hazardous to bees because they are within the bees' normal flying range.

Pesticide Drift

Pesticides don't just stick to the sprayed plant: whether in the form of liquid or dust, they usually drift downwind, especially if sprayed from a plane. Generally, it is less hazardous to apply pesticides near apiaries with ground equipment. Dr. Tew recommends that by applying pesticides in the evening or early morning when the air is calm, drift can be reduced.

Time of Application

If pesticide spraying is necessary, it should be done when there is no wind and bees are not visiting plants in the area. Some plants, such as apple trees, attract bees throughout the day, whereas others—like cucumber plants or corn—attract bees primarily in the early morning and afternoon. Dr. Tew suggests that in general, evening or early night applications are less harmful to bees than spraying in the morning or during the day.

Formulation of Pesticides

Crop dusting is usually more dangerous to honeybees and other pollinators than sprays. Wettable powders often have a longer residual effect than emulsifiable concentrates. Granular pesticides seem to present less of a hazard. Ultra-low volume formulations of some pesticides are much more toxic than regular sprays. No effective repellent has been developed that can be added to pesticides to keep bees away from treated areas.

Toxicity of Pesticides

Most agricultural pesticides have been tested for their toxicity to honeybees. However, laboratory and field results do not always agree due to peculiarities of bee behavior, length of residual life of the pesticide, or the cumulative and synergistic effects of different pesticide formulations. Farmers are urged to become experts in the effects that different pesticides have on bee communities so that they pose the least possible danger. Dr. Tew suggests the following guidelines.

- Apply pesticides only when needed.
- Use the recommended pesticide at the lowest effective rate.
- Use the pesticide least hazardous to bees that will control the specific pest. If all recommended pesticides are equally hazardous to bees, use the one that has the shortest residual effect.
- Use sprays or granules instead of dusts.
- Use ground equipment instead of aerial application to apply pesticides near beehives.
- Apply pesticides in late afternoon or at night when bees are not working the blooms.
- Avoid drift of pesticides onto plants that are attractive to bees.
- Notify beekeepers several days before applying any pesticide that is hazardous to honeybees, which will give them a chance to protect their colonies.[4]

He also recommends the following precautions for beekeepers.

- Place colonies where they will be away from fields that are routinely treated with hazardous pesticides and will not be subjected to pesticide drifts.
- Identify your apiary. Post your name, address, and phone number in a conspicuous place near your apiary. Let farmers and custom applicators in your area know where your apiaries are located so they will not unknowingly poison them.
- Be familiar with pesticides commonly used in your area and what their application dates are.
- Relocate colonies that are exposed repeatedly to hazardous pesticides. Also, remember that soon after colonies are moved to a new location, foraging bees search for water. They may collect water that has been contaminated with pesticides. To reduce the chance of bee losses, provide clean water near the hives.[5]

Creating a Welcoming Habitat
for Honeybees and Other Pollinators

Many of us live in rural or suburban areas where honeybees and other insect pollinators live. Maintaining diverse groups of pollinators is vital to a healthy environment and in protecting the human food supply.

The subject of pollination is extremely complex and several textbooks and hundreds of scientific papers have been devoted to this important topic. Detailed information about native plants in your specific bioregion that draw pollinators is available from publications like the Brooklyn Botanic Garden's acclaimed all-region gardening guides, including *Going Native: Biodiversity in Our Own Backyards, Wildflower Gardens,* and *The Wildlife Gardener's Guide* (http://shop.bbg.org). Local colleges, state and USDA Agricultural Research Service offices, and regional botanical gardens are also excellent sources for information. Yet some basic guidelines for how to create a healthy habitat for pollinating insects may be useful here.

Provide Plants for the Entire Season

Provide a range of plants that bloom in sequence from early spring until late autumn. Making sure that many different pollinators have access to blooms throughout their various flight periods will help maintain healthy pollinator populations throughout the growing season.

Go for Color and Shape

Bees have good color vision and the wonderful colors of many plants are intended to attract them, so it is always a good idea to include plants of many colors in your garden. Research has shown that bees are especially attracted to plants that are blue, purple, violet, white, and yellow.

Like humans, different types of bees and other pollinating insects are attracted to different shapes. Insects come in many different sizes and have different tongue lengths. So try to take a variety of flower sizes and shapes into account when creating your garden.

Plant Flowers in Clumps

In his paper *Plants for Native Bees,* Matthew Shepherd suggests that flowers be planted in clumps, because these are more attractive to bees than lone plants. Specifically, he suggests that clumps be at least four feet (1.2 meters) in diameter.[6]

Focus on Native Plants

Native plants are generally considered to be preferable to introduced plant species, because they help maintain a regional diversity of plants and pollinators. They are also well adapted to local conditions and require minimal attention. These would include plants that are not just native to the continent but those that are native to and genetically adapted to the local bioregion. Plus, bees seem to be more attracted to native plants than to exotic species.

Conservation or Restoration?

Environmentalists suggest that conserving existing original habitats should generally take priority over restoration. While restoration may indeed be necessary when a native habitat has been extremely degraded or destroyed, a restored habitat might not replicate every component that is important to pollinators.

Leave the Trees

Dead trees and fallen branches are traditionally important nesting places for bees and other pollinators. While many people prefer a more manicured environment—and a growing number of people are harvesting wood from fallen trees for fuel—retaining dead branches or trees is an important part of habitat management and will help maintain healthy bee populations.

Creating Bee Nesting Habitats

An increasing number of homeowners have been creating nesting habitats for bees and other insects. Drilled-board trap nests can be attached to fence posts, dead trees, or buildings.* Or, nest boxes of wood or Styrofoam

---

*For detailed instructions on making drilled-board trap nests, visit the website of either Washington State University at Snohomish (http://snohomish.wsu.edu/garden/beekeep .htm) or the National Wildlife Organization (www.nwf.org/backyardwildlifehabitat/ beehouse.cfm).

with plastic or rubber-hose entrance tunnels can be built for bumblebee species that nest underground.

Develop a Plant List

Develop a listing of native plants that will attract honeybees and other pollinators to your neighborhood. While you'll want to find out which plants are best adapted to your local bioregion, the Xerces Society for Invertebrate Conservation has provided the following partial list of native and garden plants that bees find especially attractive.

Native Plants

aster

black-eyed Susan

caltrop

creosote bush

currant

elder

goldenrod

huckleberry

Joe-pye weed

lupine

Oregon grape

penstemon

purple coneflower

rabbit-bush

rhododendron

sage

scorpion-weed

snowberry

stonecrop

sunflower

wild buckwheat

wild lilac

willow

Garden Plants

basil

cotoneaster

English lavender

giant hyssop

globe thistle

hyssop

marjoram

rosemary

wallflower

thyme[7]

Encourage Diversity

Many environmentalists are concerned that in North America humans depend wholly on *Apis mellifera,* which I mentioned earlier is not native to the Americas, to pollinate domestic crops while native bees—such as mason bees, digger bees, bumblebees, and carpenter bees—are largely ignored. Even though they are wonderful pollinators, total dependence on honeybees for pollination is harmful to the well-being of the species itself as well as to those of us who depend on honeybees to pollinate our food supplies.

To lessen the dependence of agriculture on the honeybee population Mace Vaughan, a Cornell-educated entomologist and conservation director of the Xerces Society, recommends increasing the populations of these native bee species. In an address given at the 28th annual Ecological Farming Conference held in Monterey, California, in January 2008, he recommended that farmers and gardeners encourage native bees by providing nesting sites and year-round flowers. Vaughan also suggested leaving soil untilled, minimizing pesticide use, and providing bee blocks, which are tunnels drilled into wood.[8]

Conclusion

Colony collapse disorder has shown us that the honeybee is a vital link between humans and the planet. Not only does the bee provide us with honey for food and healing—which this book has explored in great detail—but this super-pollinator also is responsible for a tremendous bounty of food, including carrots, broccoli, onions, pumpkins, apples, and blueberries, that is brought to our kitchen tables. Like the proverbial "canary in the coal mine," the threat to the survival of this tiny yet miraculous insect reveals our vulnerability as a species. This calls upon us to change how we live as citizens of this planet, and especially how we grow our food. These changes will not only protect the future for the honeybee but also will ensure the survival of the human race.

HONEY VARIETIES

The color and flavor of honeys differ depending on the nectar source (the blossoms) visited by the honeybees. In fact, there are more than 300 types of honey available in the United States alone, each originating from a different flower. The varieties of honey around the world numbers in the thousands. It's not surprising that some honey enthusiasts compare the different colors, textures, tastes, and aromas of honey to those of fine wine.

Honey color ranges from nearly colorless to dark brown, and its flavor varies from delectably mild to distinctively bold, depending on the

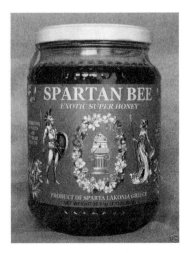

Figure A.1. Spartan Bee brand honey from Greece

plants where the honeybees obtain their nectar. Some honeys—like lavender and orange blossom—are renowned for their delicious taste, while others—such as almond—taste bitter or are otherwise unappealing. As a general rule, light-colored honey is milder in taste and dark-colored honey is stronger.

Honey is produced throughout the United States (there is even a beekeeper who has hives on the roofs of dozens of New York City apartment houses). Yet depending on floral-source location, certain types of honey are produced only in a few regions. Tupelo honey, for example, is produced mainly in northern Florida, while macadamia nut honey can be found primarily in Hawaii. Manuka honey is produced only in certain parts of New Zealand, and the sidr honey harvest is limited to parts of South Yemen. In addition to the United States, which ranks number four in honey production, the top ten honey-producing countries in the world include China (the world's largest producer and exporter), Turkey, Argentina, Ukraine, Russia, India, Mexico, Ethiopia, and Spain.

Following is a list of some of the honey varieties produced in North America and abroad. To learn more about the types of honey available in your area, contact a local beekeeper, farmers' market, beekeepers' association,

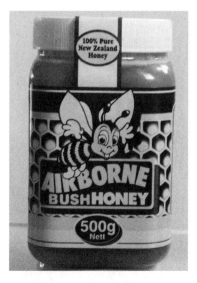

Figure A.2. Airborne Bush (forest) Honey, New Zealand

or honey packer. American readers can also consult the "Honey Locator" link sponsored by the National Honey Board (see the resources); in addition, a number of reputable companies that sell honey can be found there.

Acacia Ranging from almost transparent to light yellow in color, acacia honey is known for its pleasant fragrance and mild taste. It does not crystallize easily and is recommended as a wholesome, nutritious food. Russian folk healers use acacia honey to treat acute respiratory diseases, headaches, kidney diseases, and atherosclerosis, as well as as a sedative for nervous disorders and insomnia. Acacia honey is produced in a number of countries around the world, including the United States, Russia, and New Zealand.

Alfalfa Alfalfa honey is produced extensively throughout Canada and the United States from this purple-blossomed plant. Some varieties are light in color and feature a mild flavor and aroma, while others have a deep smooth flavor and texture that has been likened to molasses. A perfect kitchen companion, alfalfa honey is popular for cooking and baking.

Avocado Avocado honey is gathered from avocado blossoms in California, Mexico, and Chile. Avocado honey is dark in color and—like the fruit—has a rich, buttery taste.

Blackberry Wild blackberry honey is gathered in abundance from Alaska to California, although most is produced in the coastal areas of Washington state. The honey is white to extra-light amber (in some areas it is reported to have a smoky cast) with a robust yet pleasant flavor.

Blueberry Blueberry plants are especially dependent on pollination from honeybees. The nectar from the white blossoms makes a honey that is light amber in color, but with a full, well-rounded flavor. In North America blueberry honey is produced primarily in New England, Michigan, and Ontario.

Blue Borage Blue borage is a small plant commonly found in the dry wastelands of New Zealand's South Island. The honey is light pinkish brown in color with a clean taste hinting of lemon. In New Zealand blue borage honey is a popular remedy for relieving fatigue and stress.

Buckthorn   In Yemen a creamy winter honey made from buckthorn blossoms is known as bariyah honey. It has a heady floral aroma, and the taste is said to be like a mixture of butter, wildflowers, and herbs. Rare and expensive, bariya is traditionally enjoyed mostly by wealthy men from Yemen and Saudi Arabia.

Buckwheat   Buckwheat honey is dark and full-bodied. Because it contains more antioxidant compounds than most other honey varieties, it is considered one of the most medicinal honeys money can buy. It has long been an important part of traditional and folk medicine, and Russian healers recommend it to prevent and treat a wide range of health problems, including hypertension, rheumatism, scarlet fever, measles, and spotted fever. They also prescribe it for prophylaxis and treatment of blood vessels after radiotherapy and for people suffering from radiation sickness.

Though native to many parts of Europe (one of the finest buckwheat honeys I've ever tasted came from Russia), it is produced mostly in Minnesota, New York, Ohio, Pennsylvania, and Wisconsin as well as in eastern Canada.

Chestnut   Dark in color, chestnut honey has a strong aroma and somewhat bitter taste. Being a darker honey, it has a large amount of minerals and stronger antioxidant and antimicrobial properties than many other honey varieties. Traditional folk healers in Europe use it to treat diseases of the respiratory tract, alimentary canal, and kidneys; they also recommend it for symptoms of rheumatism and malaria. It is also a diuretic remedy.

Clover   Known for its pleasing, mild taste, clover is also one of the most popular honey types. Taken together, the numerous varieties of clover contribute more to honey production in United States and Canada than any other group of plants. Depending on the location and type of the clover itself, clover honey varies in color from white to light amber to amber.

Red clover, alsike clover, and the white and yellow sweet clovers are most important for honey production. Sweet clover in particular is considered an important source of medicinal honey. Sweet clover honey is also known as melitot honey. Traditional Russian healers use this honey to treat atherosclerosis of both the coronary and cerebral arteries and to lower high blood pressure. They also use it externally in the form of plasters on furuncles (boils) and in the form of compresses (with propolis) on festering wounds and cuts.

Eucalyptus   Native to Australia, eucalyptus honey varies greatly in color and flavor. It tends to have a stronger flavor than other honeys and has a slight medicinal scent. In the United States this type of honey is produced primarily in California.

Fireweed   Fireweed honey is light in color and comes from a perennial herb that is considered prime bee pasture in western Canada as well as in the northern and Pacific regions of the United States. Featuring attractive pinkish flowers, fireweed grows in the open woods and reaches a height of three to five feet (1 to 1.6 meters). It is among the first plants to grow after a forest fire.

Goldenrod   Goldenrod honey comes in a variety of colors and tastes. Many who buy this honey locally use it to resolve their allergy problems. Especially popular with mead makers, this honey tends to granulate quickly.

Hawaiian Christmas Berry   Bees gather this honey from the Christmas berry shrub (*Schinus terebinthifolia*), a native of Brazil that is considered one of the worst invasive plants in Hawaii. It has a rich amber color and a bold taste with hints of brown sugar and molasses. A study at the University of Illinois found that this honey has a very high concentration of healthful antioxidants, scoring second after buckwheat honey.

Hawthorn   Known for its bitter taste, hawthorn honey is considered wholesome and nutritious. Like the berries that come from this plant, European traditional healers recommend it for treating heart-related disorders, including poor heart rhythm, atherosclerosis, tachycardia, cardiac asthenia, and hypertension. They also recommend it for treating heightened thyroid gland function and insomnia.

Kamahi   A New Zealand native, the creamy-colored kamahi flower imparts a light amber color along with distinctive, full-bodied complexity of flavors, including what some gourmets describe as "smoky."

Lehua   This rare honey is made from nectar gathered from ohi'a trees, which grow on Hawaiian lava flows. Lehua is a water-white honey with a floral, buttery flavor. Lehua honey crystallizes quickly, making it naturally creamy.

Linden   Linden honey (also known as basswood) is produced from the blossoms of the linden tree. Water-white in color, it has a fresh lime taste and a distinctive lingering flavor. It is renowned in Europe for its sedative and antiseptic qualities.

Long'an   The long'an tree is native to southern China, but it is also found in Taiwan, Vietnam, Thailand, and other Southeast Asian countries. Long'an honey is dark in color, very sweet in taste, and has a strong, fruity flavor. It is a popular ingredient in Taiwanese-style tapioca "bubble" tea.

Macadamia Nut   Native to the Hawaiian Islands, honeybees from macadamia-nut orchards produce this sweet, flowery honey. It is reputed to be great on oatmeal, pancakes, ham, and in tea.

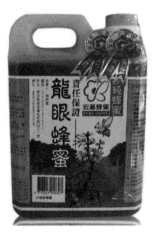

Figure A.3. Long'an honey from Taiwan

Manuka   Native to parts of New Zealand, manuka honey is dark amber in color. While not considered a gourmet honey for eating or flavoring food and drink, it is perhaps the most medicinal of honeys available. Generally speaking, the varieties with the lowest (or no) UMF rating are considered the most pleasant to eat, while those of UMF 20 or higher are considered less palatable.

May   May honey is especially popular among people living in Russia and Ukraine. It is traditionally made from the nectar of the first spring flowers, including coltsfoot, willow, and those from blooming orchards. In the middle belt of Russia, they begin to produce May honey in the second part of June. A popular medicinal honey, it is widely used to treat cough, headache, fatigue, and fever. It is also said to be useful for strengthening hair.

Mesquite   The flowers of the mesquite tree are prized by honeybees living in the American Southwest. Light in color, mesquite honey offers a lighter and sweeter taste than other honey varieties. It is often used in barbecue recipes, making it a "must-have" in many kitchen cabinets.

Motherwort   Made primarily from the nectar of a medicinal herb, motherwort honey is light gold in color and features a delicate aroma and distinctive taste. In Russia traditional healers use it to prevent and

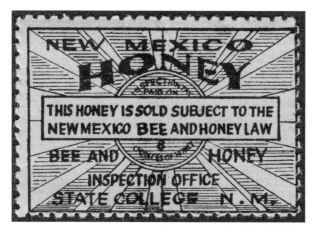

Figure A.4. Old honey inspection stamp, New Mexico

treat cardiovascular diseases and for strengthening the heart muscle. They also recommend it as a sedative and to facilitate wound healing.

Mountain   Popular in Russia, this viscous honey is usually dark yellow to reddish brown in color with a distinctive tart and bitter taste. Bees gather this honey primarily from chestnut trees, acacia, heather, citrus plants, and eucalyptus trees, as well as from the grasses of alpine meadows. Russian healers consider it effective for treating cardiovascular diseases, stress, and endocrine system disorders.

Orange Blossom   Orange blossom honey often comes from a combination of citrus sources. Usually light in color and mild in flavor, it features the fresh scent and light taste of citrus. In the United States orange blossom honey is produced primarily in Florida, southern California, and parts of Texas.

Palmetto   Saw palmetto honey is produced from North Carolina to Florida and west along the Gulf Coast to Texas. A popular table honey enjoyed primarily by locals, it has a distinctive light flavor and a light-amber to amber color.

Pohutakawa   This exotic honey comes from the nectar of the flowers of a tough, adaptable coastal tree that is commonly referred to as the New Zealand Christmas tree. The honey's color is off-white, and its aroma is one of musky damp leaves. The flavor has been described as earthy butterscotch. Because Pohutakawa honey will crystallize quickly, it is always packed as a cream rather than a liquid.

Rapeseed   A yellow flowering plant that is part of the Mustard family, rapeseed is the largest single floral source for honey production in China, and it is also an important honey source in Malaysia, Thailand, and Vietnam. Rapeseed honey is sold primarily for bakery use. Its color ranges from light amber to amber, and it has a slight peppery taste.

Raspberry   Produced from the blossoms of the wild raspberry bush, this honey is light yellow in color and has a pleasant raspberry taste. In folk medicine it is widely used to treat diseases of the upper respiratory tract, inflammation of the alimentary canal, and respiratory organs.

In addition to parts of Russia, this honey is produced primarily in the Canadian province of Quebec.

Rewarewa   Native to New Zealand, rewarewa honey comes from a bright-red, needlelike flower also known as the New Zealand honeysuckle. Its general appearance is light amber with orange hints and a flavor described as clean, sweet, smoky, and herbaceous.

Sage   Light in color, sage honey is known for its mild but pleasing flavor. It is extremely slow to granulate, making it a favorite among honey packers for blending with other honeys to slow down granulation. It is produced primarily in California, but it is also found in Europe.

Sidr   Sidr honey is produced from the blossoms of the sacred sidr, or jujube, tree, which grows primarily in uncultivated desert areas of Hadramot in southern Yemen. Considered a highly medicinal honey, it is used by traditional healers to treat liver problems, stomach ulcers, respiratory infections, digestive problems, constipation, and eye diseases. Yemeni men also mix it with carrot seeds to use as a powerful aphrodisiac. This rare honey is very difficult to find outside of the Middle East and can cost more than $200 a pound.

Sourwood   Especially popular among residents of the Appalachian Mountains from northern Georgia to Pennsylvania, honey from the blossoms of the sourwood tree has a sweet, spicy, anise aroma and flavor.

Star Thistle   Although this honey comes from a plant regarded as a troublesome weed in northern California, it is considered so delicious that people eat it by the spoonful. White to light amber in color, this mild-tasting honey is especially recommended to sweeten tea.

Sunflower   Popular in Russia, Belarus, and Ukraine, sunflower honey tends to be yellow, oily, and coarse grained. Russian folk healers recommend it to treat heart disease, bronchial asthma, alimentary canal colic, malaria, influenza, and catarrh.

Thyme   Popular in the Mediterranean from Spain to Greece, thyme honey is harvested during the summer. It has a light color very similar to orange, and the taste and aroma have been described as pungent and herbal.

Tulip Poplar   Native to the eastern United States from Georgia to New York, the tulip poplar is considered a major honey-producing tree. This honey is generally dark amber in color but has a distinctively mild flavor.

Tupelo   Highlighted in the movie *Ulee's Gold,* tupelo honey is a premium honey produced mostly in the swamplands of northwest Florida. It is heavy bodied and is usually light golden amber in color with a slight greenish cast. Tupelo honey also has a mild, distinctive, and delicious taste. Because of its high fructose content, tupelo honey tends to granulate very slowly.

Wildflower   Perhaps the most popular honey variety in the world, wildflower honey is often used to describe honey from a variety of undefined flower sources. As a result, it can vary considerably in taste, flavor, and medicinal value.

RESOURCES

The field of therapeutic honey is changing rapidly. In addition to books and online databases, there are a number of organizations devoted to honey and apitherapy. Here is a short list (which is by no means comprehensive) of these available resources.

Books

Fruitless Fall: The Collapse of Honeybees and the Coming Agricultural Crisis by Rowan Jacobson (London: Bloomsbury, 2008). A compelling and well-documented book about colony collapse disorder.

The Hibernation Diet by Mike and Stuart McInnes with Maggie Stanfield (London: Souvenir Press, 2004). American edition published by World Class Emprise. A provocative book about using honey and other foods to lose weight and gain strength.

Sweetness & Light: The Mysterious History of the Honeybee by Hattie Ellis (New York: Harmony Books, 2004). A delightful and informative history of the honeybee.

Organizations and Blogs

The Active Manuka Honey Association
P.O. Box 19348, Hamilton
www.umf.org.nz
An organization of UMF-Manuka-honey producers, AMHA develops and

maintains the UMF brand. The website includes a listing of the licensees permitted to use the UMF trademark along with their websites. In addition to honey, many of these companies sell medicinal creams and gels made with manuka honey.

American Apitherapy Society, Inc.

500 Arthur Street, Centerport, NY 11721

www.apitherapy.org

The American Apitherapy Society serves its membership and the medical profession by collecting information on apitherapy and maintaining a library for members, which contains printed information, raw data, audio-visual materials, and a database. It also informs the medical profession and the general public in matters relating to apitherapy by publishing a subscription-based journal and conducting workshops.

Apitherapy News

http://apitherapy.blogspot.com

A comprehensive and up-to-date blog about all aspects of apitherapy.

Bees for Life: World Apitherapy Network

www.beesforlife.org

Bees for Life: World Apitherapy Network is an international voluntary organization of professionals and laypeople who seek to promote the therapeutic use of bee products: honey, wax, pollen, bee bread, propolis, apitoxin (bee venom), drone larvae, and royal jelly.

Canadian Honey Council

www.honeycouncil.ca

The CHC is Canada's national organization of the beekeeping industry. The CHC is the vital link between beekeeper associations, industry, and government.

Committee for the Promotion of Honey and Health

www.prohoneyandhealth.com

Made up of members of the honey industry, health professionals, and scientists, this nonprofit group has two main goals: "To create and promote a positive Honey and Health agenda that will result in greater consumer appreciation and demand for honey nationwide and enhance the already favorable image of honey by advancing sound scientific information that underscores its healthful benefits; and to support and promote the development of quality standards from within the industry, and promote an educational campaign that reinforces the need for good science to be applied in the promulgation and establishment of standards, including realistic tolerance and testing limits." The organization sponsors an annual International Symposium on Honey and Human Health.

The Honey Association
1 Bedford Avenue
London WC1B 3AU
England
www.honeyassociation.com
The United Kingdom's honey industry's official website, compiled by the British Honey Importers and Packers Association (BHIPA).

The Honey Research Unit
The School of Science and Engineering
The University of Waikato, Hamilton, New Zealand
http://bio.waikato.ac.nz/honey
Founded by Dr. Peter C. Molan, this is an excellent resource about the medicinal value of honey and provides updates on the Honey Research Unit's research.

International Bee Research Association
16 North Road, Cardiff CF10 3 DY, Wales
www.ibra.org.uk
IBRA is a charitable organization working to increase awareness of the vital role of bees in the environment and to encourage the use of bees as wealth creators. They have an extensive library and publish and distribute books on honey and bees as well as publishing the *Journal of Apicultural Research.*

National Honey Board
11409 Business Park Circle
Suite #210
Firestone, CO 80504-9200
www.honey.com
The National Honey Board conducts research, advertising, and promotion programs to help maintain and expand domestic and foreign markets for honey. The board's work is funded by an assessment of one cent per pound on domestic and imported honey. Its goal is designed to increase awareness and use of honey by consumers, the food service industry, and food manufacturers.

The National Honey Show
www.honeyshow.co.uk/index.shtml
The website of an exciting annual event that takes place in London every fall.

Where to Find Medicinal Honey

United States
The Honey Locator
www.honeylocator.com
Sponsored by the National Honey Board, the Honey Locator offers a search engine to find suppliers of many varieties of honey in the United States. You can search by state to find an apiary near you, or you can search by honey type.

Australia
Medihoney
www.medihoney.com
Now part of Comvita, Medihoney was a pioneer in the field of honey and wound-care research.

New Zealand

Comvita

Tuaranga Rotorua Highway, Te Puke

www.comvita.com

A pioneer company selling honey and other bee products; manuka honey elixirs and first-aid creams; and honey-impregnated bandages. Visitors center.

The Honey Collection

www.honeycollection.co.nz

The Honey Collection offers a range of "Pure New Zealand Skin Care products" that has UMF-rated Manuka honey as a primary ingredient.

SummerGlow Apiaries, Ltd.

131 Richards Road, RD8, Hamilton

www.manukahoney.co.nz

Holders of the first UMF-Manuka license issued, owners Margaret and Bill Bennett offer a range of UMF-manuka honeys, creams, and lotions. They also sell a sterilized UMF-16 Manuka Honey available by mail order. The honey is in a 200-g jar and is called SummerGlow Sterilized UMF16 Manuka Honey.

United Kingdom

Beekeeping Database Resources

www.beedata.com/localhoney/index.html

This website offers a listing of United Kingdom honey producers.

NOTES

Chapter 1. Who Are the Honeybees?

1. Shaowu Zhang et al., "Honeybee Memory: A Honeybee Knows What to Do and When," *The Journal of Experimental Biology* 209 (2006): 4420–21.
2. "Communication and Recruitment to Food Sources by *Apis mellifera*," Carl Hayden Bee Research Center, Tucson, Ariz., http://faculty.ksu.edu.sa/zdaher/ling1lib/Bees%20Communication.doc (accessed on May 9, 2009).

Chapter 2. Honey: Gift of the Gods

1. *Codex Standard for Honey* (Rome: United Nations Food and Agriculture Organization, 2001), 1.
2. Ibid.
3. Peter C. Molan, "Authenticity of Honey," in P. R. Ashurst and M. J. Dennis, eds., *Food Authentication* (London: Chapman & Hall, 1996), 270–71.
4. "Honey Update" for September 2007. See "Market Updates," http://skamberg.com (accessed September 8, 2009).
5. P. R. Ashurst and M. J. Dennis, eds., *Food Authentication* (London: Chapman & Hall, 1996), 281.
6. "Honey: A Reference Guide to Nature's Sweetener" (Firestone, Colo.: National Honey Board, 2005), 5.
7. Ibid.
8. Ibid., 2.
9. S. Frankel, G. E. Robinson, and M. R. Berenbaum, "Antioxidant Capacity and Correlated Characteristics of 14 Unifloral Honeys," *Journal of Apicultural Research* 37, no. 1 (1998): 30.

10. Nathaniel Altman, *The Oxygen Prescription* (Rochester, Vt.: Healing Arts Press, 2007), 72–73.

11. Patricia E. Lusby et al., "Activity of Honeys against Medically Significant Bacteria," *Archives of Medical Research* 36, no. 5 (September–November 2005): 464.

12. D. Tonelli et al., "Honey Bees and Their Products as Indicators of Environmental Radioactive Pollution," *Journal of Radioanalytical and Nuclear Chemistry* 141, no. 2 (August 1990): 427–36.

Chapter 3. Sacred Bee, Sacred Honey

1. Rudolf Steiner, *Bees* (Great Barrington, Mass.: Anthroposophic Press, 1988), 3.

2. Henri A. Junod, *The Life of a South African Tribe,* vol.1 (New Hyde Park, N.Y.: University Books, 1962), 363.

3. Frederick J. Francis, *Encyclopedia of Food Science and Technology,* second edition, vol. 1 (New York: John Wiley & Sons, 2000), 148.

4. Eva Crane, *The Archaeology of Beekeeping* (Ithaca, N.Y.: Cornell University Press, 1983), 36.

5. Hilda M. Ransome, *The Sacred Bee* (London: George Allen & Unwin Ltd., 1937), 35.

6. K. A. Allsop and J. Brand Miller, "Honey Revisited: A Reappraisal of Honey in Pre-industrial Diets," *British Journal of Nutrition* 75 (1996): 515.

7. P. K. Skianas and J. G. Lascaratos, "Dietetics in Ancient Greek Philosophy: Plato's Concept of Healthy Diet," *European Journal of Clinical Nutrition* 55 (2001): 532–37.

8. Pliny the Elder, *Natural History,* John Bostock and H. T. Riley, eds. (London: Taylor and Francis, 1855), book 11, chapter 12.

9. Holy Bible (New York: New York Bible Society, n.d.).

10. *Encyclopedia Judaica,* vol. 18, s.v. "Honey." (Jerusalem: Keter Publishing House Jerusalem Ltd. 1996), 963.

11. Abdullah Yusif Ali, *The Meaning of the Glorious Qur'an,* vol. 1. (Cairo: Dar al-Kitab Al-Masri, n.d.), 674.

12. Eva Crane, *The Archaeology of Beekeeping* (Ithaca, N.Y.: Cornell University Press, 1983), 18.

13. Carmen Aguilera, *Flora y Fauna Mexicana* (Mexico City: Editorial Everest Mexicana, 1985), 85–86.

14. Hattie Ellis, *Sweetness & Light* (New York: Harmony Books, 2004), 121–22.

15. Bobby Lake-Thom, *Spirits of the Earth* (New York: Plume, 1997), 134.

16. John Muir, *The Mountains of California* (San Francisco: Sierra Club Books, 1989), 257–58.

17. Hattie Ellis, *Sweetness & Light* (New York: Harmony Books, 2004), 132.

Chapter 4. Honey in Medicine

1. J. H. Breasted, trans., *The Edwin Smith Surgical Papyrus,* vol. 1 (Chicago: University of Chicago Press, 1980), 487–89.

2. *Aristotle Historia Animalium,* D'Arcy Wentworth Thompson, ed. (Oxford: The Clarendon Press, 1910), book 9, chapter 40, Ff2v.

3. Eva Crane, *The World History of Beekeeping and Honey Hunting* (London: Gerald Duckworth & Co. Ltd., 1999), 503.

4. Ibid., 509

5. Peter C. Molan, "Why Honey Is Effective as a Medicine. I. Its Use in Modern Medicine," *Bee World* 80, no. 2 (1999): 80.

6. Pliny the Elder, *The Natural History,* John Bostock and H. T. Riley, eds. (London: Taylor and Francis, 1855), book 20, chapter 50.

7. Eva Crane, *The World History of Beekeeping and Honey Hunting* (London: Gerald Duckworth & Co. Ltd., 1999), 509.

8. The New Oxford Annotated Bible (New York: Oxford University Press, 1973).

9. Vaidya S. K. Shandra (Khandal), *Honey & Its Ayurvedic Approach* (Jaipur: Production Scheme, 2005).

10. Ibid.

11. Eva Crane, *The World History of Beekeeping and Honey Hunting* (London: Gerald Duckworth & Co. Ltd., 1999), 609.

12. Nigel Wiseman and Andrew Ellis, *Fundamentals of Chinese Medicine* (Brookline, Mass.: Paradigm Publications, 1995), 343.

13. Abdullah Yusif Ali, *The Meaning of the Glorious Qur'an,* vol. 1. (Cairo: Dar al-Kitab Al-Masri, n.d.), 674.

14. Hilda M. Ransome, *The Sacred Bee* (London: George Allen & Unwin Ltd., 1937), 73.

15. Ibid., 72–73

16. Eva Crane, *The World History of Beekeeping and Honey Hunting* (London: Gerald Duckworth & Co. Ltd., 1999), 511.

17. Ibid.

18. Ibid.

19. Pamela Munn and Richard Jones, eds., *Honey and Healing* (Cardiff: International Bee Research Association, 2001), 2–3.

20. "Honey As Medicine In The Middle Ages," www.honey-health.com/honey-15.shtml (accessed May 10, 2009).

21. Elias Lönnrot, *The Kalevala,* book 1, John Michael Crawford, trans. (New York: John B. Alden, 1888), 171–72.

22. Hilda M. Ransome, *The Sacred Bee* (London: George Allen & Unwin Ltd., 1937), 273.

23. Peter C. Molan, "Why Honey Is Effective as a Medicine. I. Its Use in Modern Medicine," *Bee World* 80, no. 2 (1999): 80.

24. Joe Traynor, *Honey: The Gourmet Medicine* (Bakersfield, Calif.: Kovak Books, 2002), 14.

25. H. C. A. Vogel, *The Nature Doctor* (New Canaan, Conn.: Keats Publishing, 1991), 455.

26. Miki Fukuda et al., "Jungle Honey Enhances Immune Function and Anti-tumor Activity," *eCam 2009* (January 12, 2009): 1.

27. Naomi M. Saville, "Apitherapy in Community-based Health Care in Nepal," paper for the "Hive Products" session of the 7th IBRA Conference on Tropical Bees: Management and Diversity; and the 5th Asian Apicultural Association Conference, 19–25 March 2000, Chang Mai, Thailand.

28. Eraldo Medeiros Costa-Neto et al., "Los insectos medicinales de Brasil: primeros resultados," *Boletin Entomologica Aragonesa* 38 (2006): 399–400.

29. Eraldo Medeiros Costa-Neto, "Faunistic Resources Used as Medicines by an Afro-Brazilian Community from Chapada Diamantina National Park, State of Bahia," *Sitientibus, Feira de Santana* 15 (1966): 214.

30. Eraldo Medeiros Costa-Neto and Maria Vanilda M. Oliveira, "Cockroach Is Good for Asthma: Zootherapeutic Practices in Northeastern Brazil," *Human Ecology Review* 7, no. 2 (2000): 44.

Chapter 5. How Does Honey Heal?

1. C. J. Sullivan et al., "Superbug Strikes in City," *New York Post,* October 26, 2007, p. 1.

2. Carmel Thomason, "Could This Bee How We Defeat Superbug?" *Manchester Evening News,* June 18, 2007, p. 8.

3. R. M. Klevens et al., "Invasive Methicillin-resistant *Staphylococcus aureus* Infections in the United States," *The Journal of the American Medical Association* 298 (October 17, 2007): 1763–71.

4. Arne Simon et al., "Medical Honey for Wound Care—Still the 'Latest Resort'?" *Evidence Based Complementary and Alternative Medicine* 6, no. 2 (2009): 165–73.

5. Peter C. Molan, "The Antibacterial Activity of Honey: The Nature of the Antibacterial Activity," *Bee World* 80, no. 2 (1999): 17.

6. C. H. Farr, *Protocol for the Intravenous Administration of Hydrogen Peroxide* (Oklahoma City: International Bio-Oxidative Medicine Foundation, 1993), 29–31.

7. K. Brudzynski, "Effect of Hydrogen Peroxide on Antibacterial Activities of Canadian Honeys," *Canadian Journal of Microbiology* 52 (2006): 1228.

8. Patricia E. Lusby et al., "Activity of Honeys against Medically Significant Bacteria," *Archives of Medical Research* 36, no. 5 (September–November 2005): 464.

9. Lynne M. Bang et al., "The Effect of Dilution on the Rate of Hydrogen Peroxide Production in Honey and Its Implications for Wound Healing," *The Journal of Alternative and Complementary Medicine* 9, no. 2 (2003): 267.

10. K. L. Allen, P. C. Molan, and G. M. Reid, "A Survey of the Antibacterial Activity of Some New Zealand Honeys," *Journal of Pharmacy and Pharmacology* 43 (1991): 817–22.

11. A. Tonks et al., "Stimulation of TNF-a Release in Monocytes by Honey," *Cytokine* 14, no. 4 (May 21, 2001): 240.

12. Miki Fukuda et al., "Jungle Honey Enhances Immune Function and Anti-tumor Activity," *Evidence Based Complementary and Alternative Medicine,* eCAM Advance Access published online on January 12, 2009, http://ecam.oxfordjournals.org/cgi/content/abstract/nen086 (accessed September 8, 2009).

13. Jed W. Fahey et al., "Pinostrobin from Honey and Thai Ginger (*Boesenbergia pandurata*): A Potent Flavonoid Inducer of Mammalian Phase 2 Chemoprotective and Antioxidant Enzymes," *Journal of Agricultural and Food Chemistry* 50 (2002): 7473.

14. Nele Gheldof et al., "Identification and Quantification of Antioxidant

Components of Honeys from Various Floral Sources," *Journal of Agricultural and Food Chemistry* 50, no. 21 (2002): 5870–77.

15. Ahmed G. Hegazi and Faten K. Abd El-Hady, "Influence of Honey on the Suppression of Human Low Density Lipoprotein (LDL) Peroxidation (in Vitro)," *Evidence Based Complementary and Alternative Medicine* 6 (March 2009): 113–21.

16. Peter J. Taormina et al., "Inhibitory Activity of Honey against Foodborne Pathogens as Influenced by the Presence of Hydrogen Peroxide and Level of Antioxidant Power," *International Journal of Food Microbiology* 69 (2001): 230.

17. Basil C. Nzeako and Faiza Al-Namaani, "The Antibacterial Activity of Honey on *Helicobacter Pylori*," *Sultan Qaboos University Medical Journal* 6, no.2 (December 2006), http://web.squ.edu.om/squmj/archive .asp?year=2006&panelno=0 (accessed September 14, 2009).

18. V. Mullai and T. Menon, "Bacterial Activity of Different Types of Honey Against Clinical and Environmental Isolates of *Pseudomonas aeruginosa*," *The Journal of Alternative and Complementary Medicine* 13 (November 4, 2007): 440.

19. A. J. Tonks et al., "A 5.8-kDa Component of Manuka Honey Stimulates Immune Cells via TLR4," *Journal of Leukocyte Biology* 82 (November 2007): 1147.

20. C. J. Adams et al., "Isolation by HPLC and Characterisation of the Bioactive Fraction of New Zealand Manuka (*Leptospermum scoparium*) Honey," *Carbohydrate Research* 343, no. 4 (2008): 651–59.

21. E. Mavric et al., "Identification and Quantification of Methylglyoxal as the Dominant Antibacterial Constituent of Manuka (*Leptospermum scoparium*) Honeys from New Zealand," *Molecular Nutrition and Food Research* 52, no. 4 (2008): 483–89.

22. A. Riboulet-Chavey et al., "Methylglyoxal Impairs the Insulin Signaling Pathways Independently of the Formation of Intracellular Reactive Oxygen Species," *Diabetes* 55, no. 5 (May 2006): 1289–99.

23. K. L. Allen, P. C. Molan, and G. M. Reid, "A Survey of the Antibacterial Activity of Some New Zealand Honeys," *Journal of Pharmacy and Pharmacology* 43 (1991): 821.

24. D. J. Willix, P. C. Molan, and C. G. Harfoot, "A Comparison of the Sensitivity of Wound-infecting Species of Bacteria to the Antibacterial Activity of

Manuka Honey and Other Honey," *Journal of Applied Bacteriology* 73 (1992): 388.

25. Ana Henriques et al., "Free Radical Production and Quenching in Honeys with Wound Healing Potential," *Journal of Antimicrobial Chemotherapy* 58 (2006): 773–77.

26. P. E. Lusby et al., "Honey: A Potent Agent for Wound Healing?" *Journal of the Wound Ostomy and Continence Nurses Society* 29, no. 6 (2002): 295.

27. P. C. Molan and K. L. Allen, "The Effect of Gamma-irradiation on the Antibacterial Activity of Honey," *Journal of Pharmacy and Pharmacology* 48 (1996): 1206.

28. Richard White, Rose Cooper, and Peter Molan, eds., *Honey: A Modern Wound Management Product* (Aberdeen: Wounds UK Publishing, 2005), 99–101.

Chapter 6. How Honey Treats Wounds

1. J. J. Eddy and Mark D. Gideonsen, "Topical Honey for Diabetic Foot Ulcers," *The Journal of Family Practice* 54, no. 6 (June 2005): 553–54.

2. Brandon Keim, "Honey Remedy Could Save Limbs," *Wired News,* www .wired.com/medtech/health/news/2006/10/71925 (accessed September 10, 2009).

3. Peter C. Molan, "Why Honey Is Effective as a Medicine. I. Its Use in Modern Medicine," in Pamela Munn and Richard Jones, eds., *Honey and Healing* (Cardiff, U.K.: International Bee Research Association, 2001), 6.

4. Philip G. Bowler, "Wound Pathophysiology, Infection and Therapeutic Options," *Annals of Medicine* 34 (2002): 34.

5. Peter C. Molan, "Re-introducing Honey in the Management of Wounds and Ulcers—Theory and Practice," *Ostomy Wound Management* 48, no. 11 (November 2002): 28–40.

6. Richard White, "The Benefits of Honey in Wound Management," *Nursing Standard* 20, no. 10 (2005): 57–64.

7. P. E. Lusby et al., "Honey: A Potent Agent for Wound Healing?" *Journal of Wound, Ostomy and Continence Nursing* 29, no. 6 (November, 2002): 296.

8. Val Robson, Lee Martin, and Rose Cooper, "The Use of *Leptospermum* Honey on Chronic Wounds in Breast Care," in Richard White, Rose Cooper, and Peter Molan, eds., *Honey: A Modern Wound Management Product* (Aberdeen: Wounds UK Publishing, 2005), 103–4.

9. Peter C. Molan, "Re-introducing Honey in the Management of Wounds and Ulcers—Theory and Practice," *Ostomy Wound Management* 48, no. 11 (November 2002): 36

10. Ibid., 33.

11. Ibid.

12. Ibid., 34.

13. M. A. Subrahmanyam, "A Prospective Randomised Clinical and Histological Study of Superficial Burn Healing with Honey and Silver Sulfadiazine," *Burns* 24 (1998): 157–61.

Chapter 7. The Clinical Evidence

1. "An Ancient Healing Remedy, Honey Product Restores Skin of 67-Year-Old Attorney Who Nearly Lost His Leg Because of a Huge Ulcerated Wound," News Release, North Shore University Hospital, January 8, 2009; www .northshorelij.com/template.cfm?xyzpdqabc=0&id=204&action=detail&r ef=1139 (accessed May 19, 2009).

2. S. E. Efem, "Clinical Observations on the Wound Healing Properties of Honey," *British Journal of Surgery* 75 (July 1988): 675–89.

3. V. Robson, S. Dodd, and S. Thomas, "Standardized Antibacterial Honey (Medihoney) with Standard Therapy in Wound Care: Randomized Clinical Trial," *Journal of Advanced Nursing* 65, no. 3 (March 2009): 565–75.

4. U. Yapucu Güneş and I. Eşer, "Effectiveness of a Honey Dressing for Healing Pressure Ulcers," *Journal of Wound, Ostomy and Continence Nursing* 34, no. 2 (March–April 2007): 184–90.

5. W. Phuapradit and N. Saropala, "Topical Application of Honey in Treatment of Abdominal Would Disruption," *The Australian & New Zealand Journal of Obstetrics & Gynecology* 32 (November 1992): 381–84.

6. N. S. Al-Waili and K. Y. Saloom, "Effects of Topical Honey on Postoperative Wound Infections due to Gram Positive and Gram Negative Bacteria Following Caesarean Sections and Hysterectomies," *European Journal of Medical Research* 4 (March 26, 1999): 126–30.

7. F. R. Khan et al., "Honey: Nutritional and Medicinal Value," *International Journal of Clinical Practice* 61, no. 10 (October 2007): 1705.

8. "Honey Helps Problem Wounds," *Medical News Today,* July 31, 2006, www .medicalnewstoday.com/articles/48330.php (accessed September 8, 2009).

9. Ibid.

10. V. Robson and R. Cooper, "Using *Leptospermum* Honey to Manage Wounds Impaired by Radiotherapy: A Case Series," *Ostomy Wound Management* 55, no. 1 (January 2009): 38–47.

11. B. M. Biswal et al., "Topical Application of Honey in the Management of Radiation Mucositis. A Preliminary Study," *Support Care Cancer* 11 (2003): 242–48.

12. Joy Bardy et al., "A Systematic Review of Honey Uses and Its Potential Value within Oncology Care," *Journal of Clinical Nursing* 17, no. 19 (October 17, 2008): 2604–23.

13. Richard White, Rose Cooper, and Peter Molan, eds., *Honey: A Modern Wound Management Product* (Aberdeen: Wounds UK Publishing, 2005), 116–24.

14. A. A. Al-Jabri et al., "Antistaphylococcal Activity of Omani Honey in Combination with Bovine Milk," *British Journal of Biomedical Science* 62, no. 2 (2005): 93.

15. Noori S. Al-Waili, "Topical Honey Application vs. Acyclovir for the Treatment of Recurrent Herpes Simplex Lesions," *Medical Science Monitor* 10, no. 8 (2004): MT94–98.

16. Arne Simon et al., "Medical Honey for Wound Care—Still the 'Latest Resort'?" *Evidence Based Complementary and Alternative Medicine* 6, no. 2 (2009): 165–73.

17. R. Ingle et al., "Wound Healing with Honey—A Randomized Controlled Trial," *Suid-Afrikaanse tydskrif vir geneeskunde* [*South African Medical Journal*] 96 (September 2006): 831–35.

18. J. Stephen-Haynes, "Evaluation of a Honey-Impregnated Tulle Dressing in Primary Care," *British Journal of Community Nursing* (June 2004): S21–27.

19. C. E. Dunford and R. Hanano, "Acceptability to Patients of a Honey Dressing for Non-healing Venous Leg Ulcers," *Journal of Wound Care* 13, no. 5 (2004): 193–97.

20. E. A. van der Weyden, "Treatment of a Venous Leg Ulcer with a Honey Alginate Dressing," *British Journal of Community Nursing* 10 (June 3, 2005): S21, S24, S26–27.

21. C. D. McIntosh and C. E. Thomson, "Honey Dressing versus Paraffin Tulle Gras following Toenail Surgery," *Journal of Wound Care* 15, no. 3 (March 2004): 123.

22. S. Natarajan et al., "Healing of an MRSA-colonized, Hydroxyurea-induced Leg Ulcer with Honey," *Journal of Dermatological Treatment* 12 (2001): 33–36.

23. G. Blaser et al., "Effect of Medical Honey on Wounds Colonised or Infected with MRSA," *Journal of Wound Care* 16, no. 8 (September 2007): 325–29.

24. Joe Traynor, *Honey: The Gourmet Medicine* (Bakersfield, Calif.: Kovak Books, 2002), 17.

25. Peter C. Molan, "Re-introducing Honey in the Management of Wounds and Ulcers—Theory and Practice," *OstomyWound Management* 48, no. 11 (November 2002): 37.

26. J. J. Eddy and Mark D. Gideonsen, "Topical Honey for Diabetic Foot Ulcers," *The Journal of Family Practice* 54 (June 2005): 535.

Chapter 8. Honey for Burns

1. M. Subrahmanyam, "Honey-impregnated Gauze Versus Amniotic Membrane in the Treatment of Burns," *Burns* 20, no. 4 (August 1994): 331–33.

2. M. Subrahmanyam, "A Prospective Randomised Clinical and Histological Study of Superficial Burn Wound Healing with Honey and Silver Sulfadiazine," *Burns* 24 (March 1998): 157–61.

3. M. Subrahmanyam, "Topical Application of Honey in Treatment of Burns," *British Journal of Surgery* 78 (1991): 497–98.

4. John Y. Chung et al., "Myth: Silver Sulfadiazine Is the Best Treatment for Minor Burns," *Western Journal of Medicine* 175 (2001): 205–6.

5. R. A. Cooper and P. C. Molan, "The Use of Honey as an Antiseptic in Managing *Pseudomonas* Infection," *Journal of Wound Care* 8, no. 4 (April 1999): 161–64.

6. R. A. Cooper et al., "The Efficacy of Honey in Inhibiting Strains of *Pseudomonas aeruginosa* from Infected Burns," *Journal of Wound Care & Rehabilitation* 23, no. 6 (November–December 2002): 366–70.

7. Jenny M. Wilkinson and Heather M. A. Cavanagh, "Antibacterial Activity of 13 Honeys Against *Escherichia coli* and *Pseudomonas aeruginosa*," *Journal of Medicinal Food* 8, no. 1 (2005): 100–103.

8. L. Boukraa and A. Niar, "Sahara Honey Shows Higher Potency Against *Pseudomonas aeruginosa* Compared to North Algerian Types of Honey," *Journal of Medicinal Food* 10, no. 4 (2007): 712–14.

Chapter 9. Honey and Internal Disorders

1. Department of Child and Adolescent Health, *Cough and Cold Remedies for the Treatment of Acute Respiratory Infections in Young Children* (Geneva, Switzerland: World Health Organization, 2001).

2. Ian M. Paul et al., "Effect of Honey, Dextromethorphan, and No Treatment on Nocturnal Cough and Sleep Quality for Coughing Children and Their Parents," *Archives of Pediatric and Adolescent Medicine* 161, no. 12 (December 2007): 1140–46.

3. F. K. Menshikov and S. I. Friedman, "Curing Stomach Ulcers with Honey," *Sovetskaya Meditsina* 10 (1949): 13–14.

4. V. Lievin et al., "*Bifidobacterium* Strains from Resident Infant Human Gastrointestinal Microflora Exert Antimicrobial Activity," *Gut* 47, no. 5 (November 2000): 646–52.

5. S. Kajiwara et al., "Effect of Honey on the Growth of and Acid Production by Human Intestinal *Bifidobacterium* spp.: An In Vitro Comparison with Commercial Oligosaccharides and Insulin," *Journal of Food Protection* 65, no. 1 (2002): 214–18.

6. Adel Alnaqdy et al., "Inhibition Effect of Honey on the Adherence of *Salmonella* to Intestinal Epithelial Cells In Vitro," *International Journal of Food Microbiology* 103 (2005): 347–51.

7. I. E. Haffejee and A. Moosa, "Honey in the Treatment of Infantile Gastroenteritis," *British Medical Journal* 290 (June 22, 1985): 1866–67.

8. N. al Somal et al., "Susceptibility of *Helicobacter pylori* to the Antibacterial Activity of Manuka Honey," *Journal of the Royal Society of Medicine* 87, no. 1 (January 1994): 9–12.

9. B. C. Nzeako and F. Al-Namaani, "The Antibacterial Activity of Honey on *Helicobacter pylori*," *Sultan Qaboos University Medical Journal* 6, no. 2 (December 2006).

10. R. A. Cooper et al., "Susceptibility of Multiresistant Strains of *Burkholderia cepacia* to Honey," *Letters in Applied Microbiology* 31 (2000): 20–24.

11. N. S. Al-Waili et al., "The Safety and Efficacy of a Mixture of Honey, Olive Oil, and Beeswax for the Management of Hemorrhoids and Anal Fissure: A Pilot Study," *Scientific World Journal* 2, no. 6 (February 2, 2006): 1998–2005.

12. A. N. Koc et al., "Antifungal Activity of Turkish Honey against *Candida*

spp. and *Trichosporon* spp: An In Vitro Evaluation," *Medical Mycology* (December 2, 2008): 1–6.

Chapter 10. Honey in Oral Health and Ophthalmology

1. "Breast Milk Causes More Cavities Than Cow Milk, According To New Study," *ScienceDaily,* www.sciencedaily.com/releases/2005/10/051007092923 .htm (accessed September 8, 2009).

2. Peter C. Molan, "The Potential of Honey to Promote Oral Wellness," *General Dentistry* 49, no.6 (November–December 2001): 587.

3. Sabine O. Geerts et al., "Systemic Release of Endotoxins Induced by Gentle Mastication: Association with Periodontitis Severity," *Journal of Periodontology* 73, no. 1 (January 2002): 73–78.

4. Peter C. Molan, "The Potential of Honey to Promote Oral Wellness," *General Dentistry* (November–December 2001): 586.

5. Ibid.

6. Helen K. P. English et al., "The Effects of Manuka Honey on Plaque and Gingivitis: A Pilot Study," *Journal of the International Academy of Periodontology* 6, no. 2 (2004): 63–67.

7. M. B. Sobhi and M. A. Manzoor, "Efficacy of Camphorated Paramonochlorophenol to a Mixture of Honey and Mustard Oil as a Root Canal Medicament," *Journal of the College of Physicians and Surgeons* (Pakistan) 14, no. 10 (October 2004): 585–88.

8. Peter C. Molan, "Why Honey Is Effective as a Medicine. I. Its Use in Modern Medicine," *Bee World* 80, no. 2 (1999): 88.

9. S. E. Blair and D. A. Carter, "The Potential for Honey in the Management of Wounds and Infections," *Australian Infection Control* 10, no. 1 (March 2005): 25.

10. G. K. Osaulko, ["Use of Honey in Treatment of the Eye"], *Vestnik oftal. mologii* 32 (1953): 25–36. (In Russian.)

11. V. P. Mozherenkov, ["Honey treatment of postherpetic opacities of the cornea"], *Oftal'mologicheski zhurma* 3 (1984): 188. (In Russian.)

12. H. H. Emarah, "A Clinical Study of the Topical Use of Bee Honey in the Treatment of Some Ocular Diseases," *Bulletin of Islamic Medicine* 2, no. 5 (1988): 422–25.

13. Peter C. Molan, "Why Honey Is Effective as a Medicine. I. Its Use in Modern Medicine," *Bee World* 80, no. 2 (1999): 88.

14. Ahmad Mansour et al., "Bullous Keratopathy Treated with Honey," *Acta Ophthalmologica Scandinavica* 82 (June 2004): 312–13.

15. D. G. Shengeliia, et al., ["Experimental Investigation of General Toxicology of Antioxidant Eyedrops Davicol"], *Georgian Medical News* 145 (April 2007): 88–90. (In Russian.)

Chapter 11. Honey: Safe for Infants? Safe for Diabetics?

1. Mamdouh AbdulRhman and Nermeen Tayseer, "Not Giving Honey to Infants: A Recommendation that Should be Reevaluated," *Journal of the American Apitherapy Society* 12, no. 2 (June 2005).

2. "All About Diabetes," The American Diabetes Association, www.diabetes.org/about-diabetes.jsp (accessed September 10, 2009).

3. N. S. Al-Waili, "Intrapulmonary Administration of Natural Honey Solution, Hyperosmolar Dextrose or Hyperosmolar Distill Water to Normal Individuals and to Patients with Type-2 Diabetes Mellitus or Hypertension: Their Effects on Blood Glucose Level, Plasma Insulin and C-peptide, Blood Pressure and Peaked Expiratory Flow Rate," *European Journal of Medical Research* 8, no. 7 (July 31, 2003): 295–303.

4. N. S. Al-Waili, "Natural Honey Lowers Plasma Glucose, C-reactive Protein, Homocysteine, and Blood Lipids in Healthy, Diabetic, and Hyperlipidemic Subjects: Comparison with Dextrose and Sucrose," *Journal of Medicinal Food* 7, no. 1 (Spring 2004): 100–107.

5. O. P. Agrawal et al., "Subjects with Impaired Glucose Tolerance Exhibit a High Degree of Tolerance to Honey," *Journal of Medicinal Food* 10, no. 3 (September 2007): 473–78.

6. A. Ahmad et al., "Natural Honey Modulates Physiological Glycemic Response Compared to Simulated Honey and D-Glucose," *Journal of Food Science* 73, no. 7 (September 2008): H165–67.

7. Ronald E. Fessenden, Report to the National Honey Board from the Committee for the Promotion of Honey and Health, January 21, 2008.

Chapter 12. Honey and Wellness

1. Derek D. Schramm et al., "Honey with High Levels of Antioxidants Can Provide Protection to Healthy Human Subjects," *Journal of Agriculture and Food Chemistry* 51 (2003): 1732–35.

2. "Honey and Wellness" (Longmont, Colo.: The National Honey Board, n.d.).

3. Maria Halina Borawska et al., "Influence of Dietary Habits on Serum Selenium Concentration," *Annals of Nutrition and Metabolism* 48, no. 3 (May 6, 2004): 134–40.

4. Z. Ustinol, "Honey Enhances the Production of Lactic Acid from Bifidobacteria," *Journal of Food Science* 66, no. 3 (2001): 478–81.

5. R. D. Kreider et al., "Honey: An Alternative Sports Gel," *Strength and Conditioning Journal* 24, no. 1 (February 2002): 50–51.

6. "Honey's Nutrition and Health Facts" (Longmont, Colo.: The National Honey Board, n.d.).

7. R. D. Kreider et al., "Effects of Ingesting Protein with Various Forms of Carbohydrate Following Resistance-exercise on Substrate Availability and Markers of Anabolism, Catabolism, and Immunity," *Journal of the International Society of Sports Nutrition* 4, no. 1 (November 2007): 18.

8. "Ledger Died of Accidental Overdose," *The New York Times,* February 6, 2008.

9. Mike McInnes, "Poster No. 14. Honey, Sleep and the HYMN Cycle," First International Symposium on Honey and Human Health, Sacramento, California, January 8, 2008.

10. Ibid.

Chapter 13. The Future of Honey Research

1. Ronald E. Fessenden, Report to the National Honey Board from the Committee for the Promotion of Honey and Health, January 21, 2008.

2. Interview with Dr. Noori Al-Waili, *Apitherapy News,* April 10, 2006.

3. "Waikato Honey Research Unit: Research Interests," http://bio.waikato.ac.nz/honey/research.shtml (accessed October 11, 2009).

4. *Comvita Annual Report 2009* (Te Puke, N.Z.: Comvita, 2009), 11.

Chapter 16. A Threatened Species

1. "Questions and Answers: Colony Collapse Disorder," U.S.D.A. Agricultural Research Service, www.ars.usda.gov/News/docs.htm?docid=15572 (accessed September 10, 2009).

2. Michael Pollan, "Our Decrepit Food Factories," *The New York Times Magazine,* December 16, 2007, p. 26.

3. "A Virus Among Honeybees," *The New York Times,* September 11, 2007, sec. A, p. 26.

4. Alan Fischer, "Malnutrition May Have Helped Wipe Out 750K Bee Hives," *Tucson Citizen,* January 24, 2008, www.tucsoncitizen.com/daily/local/74960 .php (accessed September 10, 2009).

5. "Cure for Foul Brood," *The Weekly Bee Journal* 20 (June 18, 1884): 389.

Chapter 17. Restore the Environment, Protect the Bees

1. Claudio Porrini et al., "Honey Bees and Bee Products as Monitors of the Environmental Contamination," *Apiacta* 38 (2003): 63–70.

2. Dean MacCannell, "Industrial Agriculture and Rural Community Degradation," in L. E. Swanson, ed., *Agriculture and Community Change in the U.S.: The Congressional Research Reports* (Boulder, Colo.: Westview Press, 1988), 15–75, 325–55.

3. Rowan Jacobsen, private communication, 17 January 2008.

4. James E. Tew, "Protecting Honey Bees from Pesticides," Wooster, Ohio: Honey Bee Lab, The Ohio State University, http://beelab.osu.edu/fact-sheets/sheets/2161.html (accessed September 10, 2009).

5. Ibid.

6. Matthew Shepherd, "Plants for Native Bees," monograph (Portland, Ore.: The Xerces Society, n.d.).

7. Ibid.

8. Madolyn Rogers, "Scientists Say Its Time to Act Now to Ward Off a Pollination Crisis," *Santa Cruz Sentinel,* January 24, 2008, p. 1.

GLOSSARY

B-lymphocytes: A type of white blood cell that helps defend the body from disease. Their primary role is to produce antibodies to combat antigens or any substance that causes your immune system to produce antibodies against it. This can include a foreign substance from the environment such as chemicals, bacteria, viruses, or pollen. It can also be formed within the body, such as a bacterial toxin or tissue cell.

bee bread: A mixture of collected pollen and nectar or honey. Bees deposit bee bread in the cells of a comb and use it as food.

bifidobacteria: A type of bacteria that that resides in the colon. Bifidobacteria help the digestion process. They are also associated with a lower incidence of allergies and are believed to prevent some forms of tumor growth. Some bifidobacteria are used as probiotics.

blepharitis: An inflammation of the eyelash follicles. It is caused by an overgrowth of the bacteria that is normally found on the skin.

cappings: A thin layer of wax used to cover the full cells of honey in the honeycomb. This layer of wax is sliced from the surface of a honey-filled comb by beekeepers during the harvesting process.

comb honey: Honey that is produced and sold in the comb.

crystallization: The formation of sugar crystals in honey that may cause it to turn solid. It is synonymous with *granulation*.

crystalluria: Crystals in the urine, which can cause irritation of the kidneys.

cytokines: Proteins that regulate both the intensity and duration of immune response.

diastase: A nutritionally valuable enzyme that breaks down starches into maltose, a sugar.

231

erythema: An abnormal redness of the skin due to capillary congestion; it is usually the result of inflammation due to allergic reaction or infection.

exudate: Moisture exuded by a wound.

field bees: These are worker bees that collect nectar, pollen, water, and propolis for the colony. They are generally two to three weeks old.

IAPV: Israeli acute paralysis virus, which is believed to be a major cause of colony collapse disorder among honeybees.

inhibine number: The degree of dilution to which a honey will retain its antibacterial activity.

invertase: A nutritionally valuable enzyme that is involved in the breaking down of sucrose into glucose and fructose.

methemoglobinemia: A blood disorder in which an abnormal amount of hemoglobin—the oxygen-carrying molecule in red blood cells—builds up in the blood.

MIC: Minimum inhibitory concentration. It is often used as a measure of a honey's ability to destroy harmful bacteria.

MRSA: Methicillin-resistant *Staphylococcus aureus* is a bacterium that is responsible for severe infections in humans. It is also highly resistant to some antibiotics.

neutropenia: A blood disorder characterized by an abnormally low number of neutrophils, the most important type of white blood cell.

neutrophils: White blood cells that fight infection.

ocelli: A "simple eye" that refers to a type of eye design or optical arrangement that contains a single lens. This type of eye is found on many insects, including honeybees.

paraffin tulle gras: A soft dressing consisting of open-woven silk or other material impregnated with a waterproof soft paraffin wax.

PEFR: Peaked expiratory flow rate is the fastest rate at which air can move through the airways during a forced expiration starting with fully inflated lungs.

phytochemicals: A wide variety of compounds produced by plants. Some of the more commonly known phytochemicals include beta-carotene, ascorbic acid (vitamin C), folic acid, and vitamin E.

pollen: The male reproductive cell bodies produced by anthers of flowers. Pollen is collected and used by honeybees as their primary source of protein.

queen substance: A perfume-like chemical signal called a *pheromone* that attracts the drones to the queen bee.

randomized controlled trial: A prospective experiment in which investigators randomly assign an eligible sample of patients to one or more treatment groups and a control group. They then follow patients' outcomes.

silver sulfadiazine: A popular topical antibacterial cream used to treat second- and third-degree burns.

skeps: Baskets made from coiled grass or straw that are used to create hives for honeybees.

swarm: Often led by an old queen, a swarm includes a large number of worker bees and drones that leaves the parent colony to establish a new honeybee colony.

super: A part of the beehive—usually a box—used for the storage of surplus honey that the beekeeper will harvest. It is normally above the brood chamber.

T-lymphocytes: A type of white blood cell that helps defend the body from disease. Their primary role is cell-mediated immunity: an immune response that does not involve antibodies, but the activation of macrophages, natural killer cells, and the release of various cytokines in response to an antigen.

tracheal mites: A microscopic internal mite that clogs the breathing tubes of adult bees, blocking oxygen flow and eventually causing their death.

varroa mites: A type of external parasite that attacks honeybees. Also known as varroa destructor.

VRE: *Enterococci* are bacteria that are naturally present in the intestinal tract. Vancomycin is an antibiotic to which some strains of *enterococci* have become resistant. These resistant strains are referred to as VRE.

waggle dance: A unique, figure-eight dance through which a forager bee can share information with her hive mates about the direction of and distance to patches of flowers yielding nectar, pollen, or both.

INDEX

Books of Related Interest

The Oxygen Prescription
The Miracle of Oxidative Therapies
by Nathaniel Altman

A Russian Herbal
Traditional Remedies for Health and Healing
*by Igor Vilevich Zevin with Nathaniel Altman
and Lilia Vasilevna Zevin*

The Shamanic Way of the Bee
Ancient Wisdom and Healing Practices of the Bee Masters
by Simon Buxton

The Acid–Alkaline Diet for Optimum Health
Restore Your Health by Creating pH Balance in Your Diet
by Christopher Vasey, N.D.

The Naturopathic Way
How to Detox, Find Quality Nutrition, and
Restore Your Acid-Alkaline Balance
by Christopher Vasey, N.D.

Food Combining for Health
Get Fit with Foods that Don't Fight
by Doris Grant and Jean Joice

Food Energetics
The Spiritual, Emotional, and Nutritional Power of What We Eat
by Steve Gagné

Traditional Foods Are Your Best Medicine
Improving Health and Longevity with Native Nutrition
by Ronald F. Schmid, N.D.

INNER TRADITIONS • BEAR & COMPANY
P.O. Box 388
Rochester, VT 05767
1-800-246-8648
www.InnerTraditions.com

Or contact your local bookseller